Carolyn Faulder is a journali̶s̶... concerns are social and health i̶s̶... to women – and the promotio̶n̶... women in every sphere of life. She has contributed to a wide variety of publications, including the major national newspapers and magazines and several medical journals. She also enjoys teaching and lecturing. Her book *Whose Body Is It? The Troubling Issue of Informed Consent* was published by Virago in 1985. Carolyn Faulder lives in London.

The Women's Cancer Book is a comprehensive and informative guide to cancers which particularly affect women. It is down-to-earth and practical, but also sympathetic to the fears and problems of cancer sufferers, their relatives and friends. Cancer is a serious illness – but Carolyn Faulder tells us how it can be cured, and gives us the encouraging message that we can help ourselves by simple preventive measures and prompt action. Even if cancer is diagnosed, changes in lifestyle and a wide variety of orthodox and complementary treatments can give us positive control of our lives. Most women will never get cancer, but every woman should read this book.

The Women's Cancer Book

CAROLYN FAULDER

Published by VIRAGO PRESS Limited 1989
20–23 Mandela Street, Camden Town, London NW1 0HQ

*A CIP Catalogue record for this book
is available from the British Library*

Printed by Cox & Wyman, Reading, Berkshire

For Clemencia Echeverria,
my mother.

Cancer is a word, not a sentence.
(Jessie Hunt, cancer survivor)

Contents

PART TWO

Other cancers affecting women

PART THREE

Your life in your hands

Acknowledgements

There are so many people who have helped me with the writing of this book, and in so many ways, that it is impossible for me to acknowledge them all individually. Some will be unaware of the impact they have made; others will perhaps not realise to what extent they have shaped my thinking. Those who have talked with me at any length about some of the topics in it may recognise their contribution although they may not always agree with my conclusions or views.

There is one exception to anonymity I must make. Dr Maurice Slevin read the manuscript with a painstaking care and attention which I greatly appreciate. I have heeded his comments and corrected errors he pointed out. Anything that remains of a controversial nature is entirely my responsibility.

Finally, and most importantly, I wish to thank the many women who have shared with me something of their experience of cancer. Some have been voices down a telephone line; others have given me their time and their confidence on one or two occasions and we have never met again; some have become friends or were close to me right from the beginning. I owe each one of you a special debt and I would like you to know that I wrote this book with your words and example always at the forefront of my mind.

Foreword

It is often said that the unknown is more frightening than the truth. This is usually true, even when one is talking about a serious illness like cancer. Cancer has always been surrounded by misconceptions, and the female cancers have more than their fair share of misinformation. For information to be helpful, it needs to be accurate and informative and delivered in a way that can be understood by a non-specialist audience.

Carolyn Faulder's new book tackles the common female cancers with unusual clarity, insight and accuracy. While much is known about women's cancers, and knowledge is increasing all the time, there are still many areas where knowledge is uncertain or controversial. In several cancers a number of options for therapy are available. This range of choices can be confusing and frightening for someone having to make difficult and crucial decisions. The pros and cons of these controversies are presented in this book in a simple, straightforward way. This should help patients and their relatives to make rational decisions at a time when rational thought is the last thing on their minds. Prevention is always better than cure, and the chapters on prevention and screening will provide the necessary information to help people decide how to approach these very important areas.

There is now a plethora of information about cancer, often written from one or other extreme point of view. This balanced and authoritative book will be of great help to people looking for a sensible approach to this vitally important area.

Maurice Slevin, MB FRCP
Chairman of BACUP
London, 1989

Introduction

Cancer leaves no one untouched. There are one million people in Britain today who have cancer, and every year there are 200,000 new patients. For some people it is enough to hear the word for their nerves to jangle and painful memories to be aroused. Most of us will know someone who has had cancer, possibly someone who is or was in a close relationship to us. Few of us can hope to escape the presence of cancer at some time in our lives.

This is a book about the way certain cancers affect women, what treatments are available and what else women can do to improve their situation. In particular it is about breast cancer, which is the most common female cancer and the major cause of premature death in women. Since I first wrote about this cancer in the mid seventies there have been some advances in treatment, but unfortunately they are not matched by corresponding improvements in the mortality figures. Indeed, quite the reverse, as this is a cancer which is on the increase. But although medical understanding of the natural history of breast cancer has not advanced significantly, there is a change for the better in the way the disease is managed.

A more humane and compassionate approach is discernible. More doctors are prepared to consider less mutilating surgery wherever possible, and there is an emergent concern about the psychological post-operative consequences of this and other cancers. The national breast cancer screening programme for women over the age of fifty, using mammography to detect very early cancers, offers a real hope that the number of deaths can be reduced, but this depends in great measure on there being a widespread uptake of the invitation. The adjuvant treatments for early breast cancer – chemotherapy for pre-menopausal women and tamoxifen for the much larger post-menopausal group – may not be ultimately curative, but they appear to be giving women longer remissions and an enhanced quality of life. At least on this side of the Atlantic there is a concern not to allow the treatment to be worse than the disease.

There are more than 200 different cancers, and women are as vulnerable to most of them as men. Cancers of the digestive organs are equally common in both sexes and take similar courses. The total female mortality figures for this group of cancers is nearly as high as for cancers of the breast and reproductive organs combined, so I would not like readers to think that by omitting any explicit mention of them in this book, I regard them as less important. This is not so, but clearly, space does not allow me a detailed discussion of every cancer, and the suggested further reading will fill in many gaps. Implicitly, they are included in part three, which is devoted entirely to sources of help and support, both interior and exterior, for any woman suffering from cancer of any kind.

I have, however, included a chapter each on smoking and malignant melanoma and written at some length on cervical cancer because these are all areas where women can do much to help themselves. Smoking is responsible for one-third of all cancer deaths – an appalling figure when we realise that this is self-inflicted destruction. I have no wish to overwhelm the smoking reader with feelings of guilt and apprehension; they are probably latent anyway and as an ex-smoker I know that evoking such responses tends to be counterproductive. The facts are alarming. Let them speak for themselves.

Malignant melanoma is increasing at a faster annual rate

than breast cancer, but its causes are not unrelated to lifestyle and fashion. We live in a perverse world where to be born brown-skinned is cause for contempt, whereas to fry ourselves brown is a matter for envy and emulation.

Cervical cancer is preventable. A simple test and, if necessary, one-stop outpatient treatment can permanently remove the problem.

For many people the reality of cancer means that they will have to learn how to live with it, perhaps for many years as a chronic disease. Although cancer can be cured – more often than most people realise – there will always be some people who are not so lucky, whose cancer returns. Five years is normally taken as a signpost for survival but the disease is capricious and it is well known that it often recurs much later. Recurrence does not necessarily spell disaster. Many people survive for years following their first recurrence; indeed, they may enjoy several good periods of remission.

Cancer patients constantly surprise their doctors by their ability to defy even the most gloomy prognosis, and treatments for secondary and advanced cancer have improved dramatically in recent years as the medical profession has begun to appreciate how much can be done to enhance the quality of life even for patients at an advanced stage of the disease. I have not had the space to discuss palliative medicine (as opposed to curative), nor have I been able to look at the work of the hospice movement in particular which has achieved so much in revolutionising medical and social attitudes to the care of the dying. However, many of the organisations listed at the end of the book concentrate most of their efforts on supporting and caring for patients with advanced cancer. I have also listed a few helpful books and a glance at their bibliographies will take the interested reader further into this area.

I have necessarily been fairly selective in my chapter references. I have chosen only to give a specific reference where I felt that the point being made or fact produced was new or controversial. This is not intended as a medical textbook but as a useful and reasonably comprehensive guide both for lay people and health professionals who may not be cancer specialists but whose work brings them into contact with cancer patients.

Since this book is published in the year of Europe against Cancer, it seems appropriate to conclude with

THE EUROPEAN TEN POINT CODE

1. Smoking is the greatest risk factor of all – smokers, stop as quickly as possible.
2. Go easy on the alcohol.
3. Avoid being overweight.
4. Take care in the sun.
5. Observe the health and safety regulations at work.
6. Cut down on fatty foods.
7. Eat plenty of fresh fruit and vegetables and other foods containing fibre.
8. See your doctor if there is any unexplained change in your normal health which lasts more than two weeks.

Specially for Women –

9. Have a regular cervical smear test.
10. Examine your breasts monthly.

PART ONE

Cancer of the breast

[1]

Bosom thoughts

ATTITUDES

It has become a truism to say that we live in a breast-obsessed society. Breasts are exalted as the epitome of all that is most feminine and desirable in a woman. Their size, their shape, their uplift, their cleavage, their presentation, with and without covering, are the subject of endless discussions, articles and pictures. Breasts are exhibited to sell anything and everything from newspapers to night storage heaters, toffees to tractors. They are the basic stock-in-trade of the adman's art and the romantic novelist's gushing pen.

No one could deny that the female bosom is exploited in our twentieth-century culture, but has there ever been a time or civilisation when it was not? Indeed, there were probably times when the exposure was even more blatant and provocative. Think back, for example, to the elegant Minoan ladies in Crete, *c.* 3000 BC, who are depicted in wall paintings in their long, elegantly pleated dresses with the bodice cut right away to reveal their pert, pointy breasts. There has never been a time or a place when men have not been fascinated and enchanted by the female bosom. They have sought to reproduce its curving beauty in a variety of ways and for a variety of reasons – religious, sexual and artistic – not only by straightforward imitation but by suggestion in the shape of their artifacts and even their weapons. Pots, vases, bowls, shields and helmets all reflect the rounded female breast. Look around you and you will see many other man-made objects, ancient and modern: some created for worship, others for aesthetic pleasure, some purely functional, but all evoking these sensuous generous contours. No doubt if we were to count them all up there are probably at least as many breast images in the world around us as those which reflect the phallic shape.

Fashion, recorded through paintings and other visual media, tells us a good deal more about the way people actually lived and thought than many a historian's chronicle. Looking at the records earlier civilisations have left us, there seem to be few periods when the bosom was not, quite literally, prominent.

The late James Laver, a fashion historian of some wit and discernment, suggested that the clothes we wear unconsciously reflect our attitudes to the opposite sex.[1] Most of human history has been dominated by patriarchal societies, so men have dressed on the class-conscious 'hierarchical principle' – on the whole formally and pompously – to impress, on the one hand, their male rivals with their importance; and, on the other, the women they sought to win by their status and their capacity to provide. Women, for their part, having almost always had to rely on their looks and powers of attraction to acquire a man, a home, security and minimum respect, have dressed alluringly, embodying the sex-conscious 'seduction principle'.

Calculated exposure is the basic feature of this principle, but since men are easily bored, the focus has constantly altered. Bosoms, legs, ankles, feet, wrists, shoulders, necks, waists – every tiny portion of the female anatomy has been the object of male lustful interest at one time or another, constituting what the psychologist J. C. Flugel calls 'the shifting erogenous zone'. The more prudish the society the more susceptible, apparently, it becomes to titillation and temptation. It is not altogether fanciful to find something in common between the Victorians who were so shocked by the mention of legs that they felt compelled to cover even the

inanimate ones supporting their pianos and today's funda-
mental Muslims who have driven their young educated
women back into the *chador*.

Bosoms, however, have been more constantly erogenous
than most. Even during periods when religious taboos have
been at their height, men and women have found ways of
evading moral disapproval, like the Renaissance painters who
would use their beautiful mistresses as a model for the Virgin
Mother tenderly offering her perfect breast to the Holy Infant.

Laver also pointed out that whenever women have achieved
a measure of emancipation, their clothes correspondingly
reflect an indifference to male approval. Instead they dress to
please themselves, which may be either comfortably or
'shamelessly'. Writing in the fifties and sixties, he believed
that the process of change towards female emancipation had
become irreversible; hence the dominance of the 'utility
principle' where, neither sex needing to impress the other,
dress becomes androgynous.

His theory could explain another characteristic of our
modern Western society which finds expression in the crudely
commercial exploitation of women's bodies, and particularly
their breasts, sometimes to the point of freakishness. Could
this be man's way of exacting his revenge for woman's escape
from his control? Or maybe it is because men have never
outgrown their childish awe of the big-bosomed earth
mother, nor perhaps found new sexual outlets to compensate
for their sense of loss which makes so many of them project
their unsubtle fantasies into every facet of our day-to-day
lives. Whatever the reason, the fact is that, pleasurably or
not, we are obliged to swallow big boobs with our morning
juice, see them bending over us in gross outline from the
hoardings as we travel to and from work, and find it
impossible to avoid their insistent presence as we read our
newspapers, flick through magazines, look at a film or watch
television.

The child begins its life at its mother's breast and never
entirely loses its need for the warmth, comfort, nourishment

and sensual delight that it offers. If the child grows into a woman she can enjoy the pleasure of offering her own breasts to her lover and to her child, but a boy grown into a man must find other women to replace the first woman in his life. Sometimes a man can be so jealous of his wife's breasts that he doesn't want to share them with his child. He may use as justification the excuse that breastfeeding will ruin their shape, but what he really resents is someone sharing his toys and taking time and attention away from him.

Sadly, some women feel ashamed of their breasts when they become swollen and veined with milk. They fear that the maternal function so obviously taking over from the sexual will repel their partner. Some men, it is true, do react in this way. If this is a problem in your relationship, try to talk through these negative feelings together, because it seems a great shame to allow them to prevent you from enjoying the delights and advantages of breastfeeding.

A woman's attitude to her body, and to her breasts in particular, is influenced by so many different strands in her environment; the society in which she lives; the family upbringing she has had; the cultural orthodoxies she has accepted and the self-image that she has been encouraged to foster. The link between body image and sense of self-esteem is very close. If you feel good inside your skin, and if you feel happy about the way your body functions and how it appears to others, then your positive self-appreciation will be reflected in a strong, confident self-identity.

Women may complain at the way men make capital out of their bodies, but are they so blameless themselves? Exploitation will certainly never cease until women themselves stop conniving at it. Just by thinking in the male terms of 'under-privileged' and 'well-endowed', a woman is denying scientific evidence and her own experience, which tell her that size and shape have little to do with sexual gratification and are most unlikely to affect her ability to breastfeed, should she want to. Yet what woman has not lamented and agonised at some time in her life about her breasts: they developed too early or too late; she thinks they are too big or too small, not round enough or too saggy. A woman rightly feels that her breasts express something of her essential femaleness, and the man who loves her will support her in that belief. But always remember that your breasts are only a part, never the whole, of what makes you a woman.

FACTS

The human breast is a paired mammary gland which first appears as a minute swelling in the six-week-old foetus. By the time the child is born, boy and girl alike, it will have an elementary internal system of large milk-ducts and, externally, two nipples each surrounded by a small circle of deeper pink which is called the areola. The breasts remain flat in both sexes until puberty.

When a girl reaches this stage of development, usually between the ages of eleven and thirteen, she starts secreting the hormones oestrogen and progesterone. These cause many changes in her body, preparing her for her adult role of reproduction. The most obvious external change, together with growing body hair in the genital area and under-arm, is her developing bosom. The areola swells slightly while the ducts begin to grow internally, branching out into smaller ducts which end in tiny milk-producing glands. Each of these ducts is contained in lobular segments of tissue which are embedded in fat and separated from each other by fibrous tissue. The ducts converge, like the spokes of a wheel, on to a central reservoir just behind the areola where the milk collects when a woman is lactating (producing milk) after childbirth. There may be anything from twelve to twenty lobules in the breast, and each has its own fine opening through the nipple. As the adolescent girl grows into a fully adult woman these lobular structures develop further and more fat accumulates, giving the young female breast its characteristically round, firm shape. The size of the breast depends on the amount of fatty and fibrous tissue, not on the glandular element, which is concentrated in the central and upper part.

The breast tissue is attached to the underlying pectoral (chest) muscles and the overlying skin by fine ligaments. Sometimes these strands, which are called Cooper's ligaments, become invaded by tumour and contract, causing the skin covering the breast to appear dimpled or puckered. The breast is basically hemispherical, but it does have a tongue-like extension leading into the armpit; this is called the tail of the breast or the axillary tail.

Axilla is the medical term for armpit and it is a word to remember, because it occurs frequently in this book to describe the position of certain very important lymph nodes. The lymph nodes are small masses of gland tissues all over the body through which lymph, a colourless fluid similar to blood but without the red corpuscles, drains and is purified. They are a vital part of the body's defence mechanism against disease and they are discussed in more detail in chapters 6 and 9. In the breast area there are, in addition to the axillary nodes, the pectoral nodes which run behind the breast and up the outer side, the subclavicular nodes just below the collarbone, and the internal mammary nodes which run in a chain between the two breasts.

Unfortunately, breasts give trouble as well as pleasure. Subject to endless hormonal assaults from puberty onwards, they are frequently sore and tender and, in some cases, extremely painful for years on end without relief. Pain does not automatically signify something sinister – indeed, quite the contrary, as cancer usually makes its first appearance in the breast without this warning – but you should *always* consult a doctor if you have persistent pain.

This part of the book is about understanding and coping with the darker side of having breasts, which threatens any woman of any age.

Why do women get breast cancer?

If that question could only be answered, we might by now have a cure for women's most lethal cancer. Breast cancer accounts for 20 per cent of all female cancer deaths and it is the main cause of women's premature death between the ages of thirty-five and sixty-four. Despite years of intensive research, a conclusive answer still eludes the scientists and epidemiologists.

Apart from not knowing what causes breast cancer, there are still many serious question marks hanging over the nature of the disease. Why, for instance, does it have so many different manifestations, and why does it so often follow an unpredictable course and outcome? Paradoxically, some women who appear to have the least favourable prognosis because they have a large tumour at the time of diagnosis, and evidence that their disease has already spread from the breast, may yet live many years longer than women diagnosed with what seems to be a small, contained 'early' tumour. Why, too – and even though it has been possible for some years now to identify certain high-risk groups – is it in general still impossible to predict with any degree of accuracy who is most likely to contract the disease?

These are the questions medical science is desperately seeking to answer. Great Britain holds the unenviable record for being top of the league (proportionate to population) for incidence. Over the past thirty years there has been a small but discernible increase in the numbers of women contracting breast cancer and it occurs mostly in the older age groups (fifty plus). The only age group for whom the incidence has actually slightly decreased is women under the age of forty-four.

The figures tell a dismal tale. In 1987 one woman in twelve developed breast cancer (in 1977 it was one in seventeen). In 1987, 15,073 women died of breast cancer (in 1977 it was 11,820). The only ray of hope lies in the survival rates, which tend to be better than for most other women's cancers and have improved marginally in recent years. This may be due in part to earlier detection, in part to the development of better, more effective treatments.

The most reliable recent statistics,[1] which take 1981 as the date of first diagnosis, show that 62 per cent of women with breast cancer can now expect to live beyond five years. This does not mean, however, that after five years without recurrence a woman has a 'chance of living indefinitely', as one breathless reporter in *The Times* would have it; merely that she has a better chance of ultimately dying from something other than her original breast cancer.[2] However, it is estimated that about two-thirds of the women who develop breast cancer will eventually die of it, and the disease has occasionally been known to recur as long as twenty to twenty-five years after the first diagnosis.

Incidentally, men can get breast cancer too. One in every 100 cases is male; he is often elderly and only rarely younger than forty. The tumour is usually central, close to the nipple, and treatment is along the same lines as for women.

Epidemiology is the name given to the scientific study of disease in the community. As in most other medical disciplines, epidemiologists tend to specialise in a particular disease – or epidemic, as the name suggests. Since most of the latter have either been vanquished or brought under control, the modern epidemiologist's area of interest has widened, and so also have the terms of reference.

The epidemiologist aims to discover the causes (aetiology) of a particular disease, thereby hoping to gain an understanding of its natural history – why it progresses and behaves in the way it does – and to use these answers to assist other researchers who are concentrating their efforts on finding a cure. To do this it is necessary to examine all possible significant factors such as the distribution of the disease, whereabouts in the world it is most prevalent and among what populations. Further investigations will include establishing whether it is age- or sex-linked, or both; whether there seem to be certain high-risk characteristics and high-risk groups; whether it appears to be genetic, environmental, viral or degenerative in origin, or possibly a combination of some or all of these, in which case it will be termed multifactorial.

The good epidemiologist is rather like a sleuth. He or she combines infinite patience with an inexhaustible capacity for detailed analysis while sifting through a mass of evidence, looking for clues. The most brilliant exponents of this science are the Sherlock Holmes or Miss Marple of the medical profession, because from analysis they move to synthesis and thence to formulating a hypothesis valid enough to merit being tested. The stories of how diseases like tuberculosis, smallpox and polio have been tracked and eventually conquered make thrilling drama; in the second half of this century, cancer – and now AIDS – offer the greatest challenge to epidemiological skills. Often a cure will come first, but until the causes are discovered there is no chance of preventing a disease.

CLUES TO CAUSES

In breast cancer there are now several important clues which are being followed up. Among the most significant are those relating to a woman's reproductive history, because they indicate that hormones – and in particular an excess of oestrogen – have an important influence.

Favourable factors include having a baby in your teens (less than one half the risk of the general population); having a delayed onset of periods (starting at fifteen rather than thirteen or younger); having an early menopause (at forty-five rather than fifty-five); keeping slim and active; and having no family history of breast cancer. It used to be thought that having several babies and breastfeeding them were also protective factors, but later studies have shown these to be of no significance either way.

Unfavourable factors are the reverse of the above: having an early menarche (first menstruation) or a late menopause (change of life), either or both of which mean that the breasts are submitted to more oestrogen cycles; having your first baby after the age of thirty-five or being nulliparous (having no children at all). As long ago as 1713 an Italian physician, Ramazzini, observed that nuns were more prone to breast cancer than their married sisters.

Demography, ethnic origin and diet

Other factors which must be taken into account when assessing a woman's vulnerability to breast cancer are where she lives and who she is. North American and West European women are the most prone, whereas if you are an Asian or a black African the likelihood is reduced dramatically. Furthermore, the disease appears to be less aggressive in Asian and African countries. An interesting fact which epidemiologists have observed for some time, but which continues to puzzle them, is that whereas Japanese women living in Japan are the least likely to develop breast cancer, their risk increases as soon as they emigrate to North America and by the third generation they are as vulnerable as their Western sisters.

The change to a high-fat diet has been suggested as at least a contributing cause, but as yet there is no conclusive evidence to support this view. However, it is certainly true that overweight women of any age are known to be at increased risk. One theory is that a high-fat calorific diet may cause changes in the structure of the breast, leading to cancer.

A new line of research suggests that there may also be a link between chronic constipation and breast cancer, possibly due to bacteria acting on food in the constipated bowel to transform ordinary cells into cancer cells. It is known that bacteria in the bowel produce female hormones, especially in women eating a lot of meat and animal fats. Constipation may cause these superfluous hormones to be reabsorbed and stimulate the growth of breast cancer cells.

Age and family history

A woman's age is the most significant risk factor. Before the age of thirty she is highly unlikely to develop breast cancer, even if she has a history of producing lumps (which, none the less, she should always refer to her doctor). But as she moves into her late thirties and forties and approaches the menopause, the risk grows and thereafter increases steadily as women go through the menopause and emerge into the later non-fertile part of their lives. There is undoubtedly a biological difference in the disease between pre- and post-menopausal women, which is confirmed by the fact that different treatments work better for the two age groups, but no one is yet certain of its precise nature.

It is now quite clear that breast cancer does run in some families, as do certain other diseases. A woman whose mother, sister or aunt developed breast cancer *before* the age of fifty has a greatly increased risk of developing the disease herself. It goes up to one in four, compared with the national average of one in twelve, and may rise as high as one in two if she is unfortunate enough to have more than one close female relative who developed the disease *before* the menopause. The risk reduces correspondingly (to one in eight) if the relative got breast cancer after the age of fifty and as the woman herself becomes older. These high-risk women do not directly inherit the disease but they do acquire a genetic predisposition to its development, possibly through the transmission of a single breast cancer gene. (See Resources for details of a special screening service for such women.)

The scientists are now on the track of this specific oncogene, a cancer-causing gene, which may not be confined to women who belong to the particular high-risk group described above. How precisely it works is still not fully understood, but its effect is to overstimulate breast tissue, causing the cells to grow and subdivide uncontrollably into a malignant tumour. Here, unravelling the mechanism of change back to its cause is very important, because only when that is understood will doctors be able to start thinking about appropriate treatments: either to stop the gene working its mischief in the first place, or to devise more effective methods of dealing with the resulting tumour.

Another high-risk group are women who have already had cancer in one breast or in some other part of the body. It seems also that as women get older, those who suffer a certain type of benign breast disease called, variously, fibrocystic disease or chronic cystic mastitis may run an extra risk. (In medical terms, a benign disease is one producing growths or a tumour which may mimic cancer symptoms but is not malignant). Recent research has, however, come up with the good news that the real risk of developing breast cancer for women in this group is confined to a single-figure percentage, about 4 per cent, and applies only to those whose breast lumps proliferate – spread and grow – and at some stage indicate atypical but non-cancerous changes in the cell structure.

Hormones

In our present state of knowledge it is still unwise to be too categorical about trying to rank these risks in their order of importance, especially as they are likely to work in combination rather than singly, but everything points the strongest finger of suspicion at hormones. So far we have discussed the possible effect of *endogenous* hormones (those produced internally by the ovaries and certain glands), but if they are as important as the evidence suggests, it follows that we should also be considering the effect of *exogenous* hormones (those administered externally). This means that the contraceptive pill, the oestrogen given in hormone replacement therapy (HRT) during and after the menopause, and hormones administered for other reasons such as averting a miscarriage, preventing lactation or aborting very early an unwanted conception (the 'morning after' pill) should all be looked at much more closely for any possible link with breast cancer. Oestrogen of itself, whether synthetic or natural, does not cause cancer, but under certain conditions – too much or in combination with other factors – it does seem able to create a receptive environment for the growth of cancer cells.

Before the menopause

The Pill was launched upon the world in the early sixties with a minimum of pre-clinical testing, a situation which would be quite unthinkable today. Soon enough, despite the heady praises for its apparently liberating effect on women's sexual lives and the ease with which it could be taken, doubts began to assail some of the more cautious members of the medical profession as they observed its other, far less pleasant consequences. An increase in vascular disease – thrombosis, strokes, varicose veins and other changes in the veins and arteries – was noticed early on. Migraines, depressions, intensified and prolonged pre-menstrual tension, weight gain, loss of libido, changes in skin pigmentation and a whole host of unexplained allergies are other symptoms which are too often dismissed by doctors as either neurotic complaints or of little significance compared to what they take to be the matter of overriding importance: not allowing their patients to become pregnant.

Today, even the Pill's most enthusiastic supporters are

forced to concede that it is the source of more than one hundred metabolic changes, many carrying long-term implications which are still not fully understood. Dr Ellen Grant, whose book *The Bitter Pill* is a sustained but well-documented attack on oral contraceptives, points out that reducing or changing the dosage provides no real safeguard against side-effects induced by metabolic changes since each woman reacts differently, depending on individual variations in her enzyme levels. (Enzymes act as catalysts, speeding up chemical reactions in all the body's organs.) She also emphasises that since hormones are known to have a profound effect on our immune system, tinkering about with them is not something to be lightly undertaken.

A zealot turned agnostic – she began her professional life as a keen researcher on the first major British trial of the Pill, but became progressively disenchanted and dismayed as she observed the results in patients – Dr Grant is better placed than most to take an informed view of its long-term effects. Her judgement is damning. She sees no virtue in its convenience but much danger in its promotion as a first-choice contraceptive, or as a means to regularise the menstrual cycle in young girls. Were it not for the consistently high dropout rate, she maintains, we would now be seeing 'an epidemic of Pill deaths'.

'It is my experience', she writes, 'that it is the stalwarts who stay on the Pill, those women who are superstrong and can withstand the steroid onslaught for much longer than women whose bodies have reacted fast and stopped them from endangering their health with oral contraceptives. I believe it is this fact which will always give an unbalanced picture in the results of trials, for they will be studying many women whose health is basically sound, and who have excellent defence systems.'[3]

So what about breast cancer? For quite a while it was thought that the Pill had a positively protective effect against breast cancer, a view based on studies showing that women who use the Pill for two or more years appear less likely to develop benign breast disease. But, points out Dr Grant, it's all a matter of how you choose to interpret the evidence. In fact, what happened was that women developing benign breast disease did so within a year of taking the Pill and immediately came off it. Less susceptible women who remain free of these and other symptoms are more likely to continue, not realising that in so doing they may be increasing their risk of cancer.

The controversy continues. Currently there are several ongoing large-scale studies looking at the Pill in relation to various cancers. Two in Oxford, headed by Professor Martin Vessey, still have many years to go before they can provide us with definitive answers. Since it is a well-known fact that carcinogenic agents can be latent for up to twenty, even thirty years, it is essential for the epidemiologists to scrutinise a whole generation of long-term Pill users. Their research is complicated by many factors, not least the changing pattern of Pill use and the changing types of Pill that have been used over the past two decades.

The Vessey study is looking at 17,000 women. An even larger study, run by Dr Clifford Kay for the Royal College of General Practitioners, is comparing 47,000 women divided equally into Pill users and a control group of non-Pill users. Dr Kay and his team have recently published their report on the first twenty years; this contains some disturbing findings, relating to both breast and cervical cancer.[4] The most significant fact about breast cancer is that younger Pill users, specifically those between thirty and thirty-four years old, are three times more likely to develop the disease than women of the same age who have never been on the Pill. Dr Kay would like to continue this study for at least another five years to see whether he can discover the reason for this. Is it because the Pill accelerates the disease – in other words causes it to occur earlier in women who would otherwise anyway have developed it at a later age – or does it actually induce an increased risk for all women taking it throughout their lifetime? Either way the implications are devastating but he needs time to monitor his groups through the menopause before he can hope to come up with more definitive answers.

Even more recently – indeed, just as this book was going to press – the results of an important controlled study based on case notes and one-to-one interviews with 755 Pill-using women – all of whom had been diagnosed with breast cancer before the age of thirty-six – and their randomly selected matched controls, were published in *The Lancet*.[5] These findings confirm quite conclusively that young women who have been on the Pill for four or more years run a significantly increased risk of developing breast cancer, irrespective of whether they have had a full-term pregnancy. The order of risk is one in 350 for women who have been on the Pill for four years or longer, going up to one in 300 for those who have been on it for more than eight years. This compares with the normal average risk of one in 500 for this age group. There is some evidence (only 'marginally significant' according to the researchers) to show that there is less risk attached to a lower-dose oestrogen Pill and that there may even be some protective effect from using a progestogen-only Pill. What they cannot be sure of at the moment is whether the increased risk from the Pill is related only to a particular form of breast cancer affecting younger women or whether it carries on as they grow older – in which case the situation would be (to quote Professor Julian Peto, one of the authors of the study) 'extremely worrying'. The same research group is now carrying out a similar study on women aged thirty-six to forty-five to try and find the answers. Meanwhile, 'women who are not having intercourse should stop taking it' [the Pill], warns Clair Chilvers of the Institute of Cancer Research, another of the authors.

So what are we to think – and, more importantly, what should we do now? As long ago as 1983, in an issue which contained two disturbing papers suggesting links between the Pill and cancers of both breast and cervix, *The Lancet* issued this warning: 'The growing evidence that the Pill has residual and long-term effects on health needs to be taken seriously and discussed rationally. It should not be dismissed or belittled because of the anxiety that might be created in the short term.'[6] When I interviewed Professor Vessey some years ago for the first edition of this book he cautiously proffered this view: 'I find it hard to believe that the Pill has no effect on the disease. It seems biologically highly improbable. The possibility of a hazardous effect in women otherwise at high risk is particularly worth watching.' In a recently published overview of contraception, which included a major section on the effects of the Pill, the author noted that the findings on breast cancer were contradictory and that the American FDA (Food and Drugs Administration) has 'encouraged further research in this area to clarify the inconsistencies in the data obtained so far.'[7]

All the same, we now have enough evidence to put us on guard. The medical attitude has been consistently to play down adverse reports on the Pill, regarding them as relatively unimportant compared to the danger of causing a flood of unwanted pregnancies. Women, the consumers of the Pill, should be aware of these findings in order to weigh up the pros and cons for themselves. Even if the risk appears negligible to the experts, we should know that it exists and decide for ourselves whether we want to take it or opt for a different method of contraception. We cannot afford to let others, however well-meaning, take such important decisions affecting our health, possibly our lives, on our behalf and without consulting us.

Meanwhile, it seems quite wrong that Dr Kay's study is currently under threat because the Medical Research Council is withdrawing funding, which means that unless Dr Kay can find money from other sources – possibly the pharmaceutical companies – it will be closed before it has achieved its aim of tracking a generation of Pill users. A second, similarly important RCGP study, planned for 120,000 women over ten years to look at the combination of changing patterns of use and user (now overwhelmingly

young single women on lower-dose pills), has also foundered
for lack of funds from the MRC at the very last moment.
This is particularly frustrating because the chop fell after
three years of careful preparation and collaboration between
Dr Kay's team and their American colleagues at the National
Institutes of Health.

Given that breast cancer is, to a great extent, hormone-
dependent, I believe that until the Pill gets positive clearance
it is only sensible to keep it under lively suspicion. As I said
at the beginning of this chapter, there are too many serious
questions still unanswered.

The menopause and after

The picture is almost as baffling when one looks at women
on the far side of fifty, mainly because so little has been done
in the way of sustained investigation into the relationship
between HRT and breast cancer. In the United States, where
many more women for very much longer have been taking
oestrogen for menopausal symptoms – and often for years
afterwards, in pursuit of the Feminine Forever dream – a
definite causal connection has been established for endometrial cancer (see page 146). Up to now nothing so clear-cut
has emerged about breast cancer. It does, however, appear
that women who use these oestrogens for more than four
years run a significantly greater risk of developing benign
breast disease.

HRT is undoubtedly an excellent therapy for women who
suffer from distressing or uncomfortable menopausal symptoms like hot flushes or vaginal dryness. It definitely has a
beneficial effect in reducing thinning of the bones (osteoporosis), providing it is taken early enough, during and after
the menopause. It is possible that it may also lessen the risk
of heart disease, although the evidence for this is conflicting.
As with the oral contraceptive, there are several variations of
hormone dosage and it should be carefully prescribed and
monitored by your doctor to meet your individual needs. But

don't get carried away with unrealistic expectations of a wonder drug to maintain you in a state of eternal youth and beauty, or fall for the line that it is a 'universal preventative medicine', as one leading British specialist was pleased to call his lecture on HRT in a conference discussing modern approaches to health promotion.[8]

Approximately 20 to 25 per cent of women are lucky enough to sail through the menopause with minimal symptoms, so they have no need to take HRT unless they want to take it as a precaution against osteoporosis. It is positively contra-indicated for women who have had cancer of the breast, ovaries or endometrium; women who have a family history of breast cancer or any kind of benign breast disease should consider it with caution.

Radiation

It is well known that excessive doses of radiation are carcinogenic. Evidence for this in relation to breast cancer is incontrovertible and comes from three sources. First, there is the aftermath of Hiroshima. An abnormally high number of Japanese women who were between fourteen and nineteen when the bomb was dropped developed breast cancer ten to fifteen years later – a particularly cruel irony in view of their normally low susceptibility. The other two groups known to be breast cancer victims of radiation are women who were exposed to large doses of X-rays as a result of treatment for tuberculosis or for chronic mastitis in the days when the potential risks were still not appreciated.

This is not a reason to be afraid of having a mammogram, which now provides the most useful screening method we have for breast cancer and diagnosis. (It is described in detail in chapter 4). The radiation dose has been reduced to the lowest degree possible. Nor should you be worried about accepting radiotherapy, either as an alternative to surgery or as an adjuvant therapy. X-ray treatments are now regulated and monitored with a fine degree of precision.

OTHER POSSIBILITIES
Personality

From earliest times, people have speculated as to whether cancer could be activated by psychological factors. Galen, a Greek physician, divided women into melancholic and sanguine types. The former, who were said to suffer from 'an excess of bile', were the ones most likely to develop breast cancer. More pertinently, he observed that regular menstruation kept women healthy and that most breast tumours developed after the menopause.

The idea that there could be a cancer-prone personality – a 'Type C' analogous to the striving, competitive 'Type A' who has been defined as high-risk for heart attack – has always had a certain popular appeal, but until recently it has been based on no measurable evidence. There have now been several studies – most notably in this country those conducted by Tina Morris and Stephen Greer at King's College Hospital, London – which do suggest that there is, if not an invariable causal connection, certainly a not infrequent relationship between particular psychological traits and breast cancer.[9]

Between 1973 and 1974 a total of 160 women admitted for biopsy because of a lump in the breast were put through exhaustive personality and life-history questionnaires; their answers were then checked out with husbands or close relatives. Of these women, sixty-nine turned out to have breast cancer and the remainder had benign disease. Stress, depression, an introverted rather than extroverted personality -- all factors which have been suspected to have a connection with cancer – appeared to be unimportant, but women with 'an abnormal release of emotions' were much more frequent in the breast cancer group. These were mainly women who tended to bottle up their feelings. Most said that they could remember losing their temper only once or twice in their lives, and some were positive that they had never done so. A smaller group of women, also with breast cancer, admitted to losing their temper at least once a month and generally being much more emotional. The women with benign disease appeared more moderate – 'apparently normal', as the researchers are careful to define it – in the expression of their emotions.

These findings are supported by another researcher, Jennifer Hughes, a psychiatrist at the University of Southampton, who has carried out similar studies with both lung and breast cancer patients. She too has found that patients with benign breast disease are more able to act assertively and to admit to feelings of hostility. Her book *Cancer & Emotion – Psychological Preludes and Reactions to Cancer* (see Resources) is a useful compendium of all the research in this field, and I will be making further reference to it.

Her summary of the typical cancer patient who emerges from these studies describes someone who is 'pleasant, unemotional, stable and calm' – a little inhibited, perhaps? – anyway, the sort of person who does not complain easily and is stoical about pain. One hesitates to make too much of such findings for fear that people will identify with the profile and immediately classify themselves as high-risk. Think about it. We have surely all known people with cancer who do not conform in any way to this description. Probably the safest conclusion to draw is that a certain type of personality does not of itself *cause* cancer, but it is just possible that when combined with certain physical conditions it can become a predisposing factor.

Stress

Several studies have attempted to show a relationship between severe stress, or a deeply felt loss – such as the death of a spouse, a child or perhaps a job – and the onset of cancer. Scientists are hesitant to accept them as more than interesting speculations because by their very nature they are difficult to prove. For one thing, different cancers have different causes, frequently more than one; for another, a distinction has to be made between what is responsible for initiating a cancer and what makes it flourish. Furthermore, the long latent period characteristic of cancer makes it impossible to pinpoint precisely when it might have started. However, there is now conclusive laboratory evidence to show that traumatic events like bereavement or divorce do exact a physical toll; our hormones and our immune defences can be affected quite dramatically.

Since people differ so widely in their ability to handle stress, it is highly likely that they are equally variable in their susceptibility to disease. It is, therefore, probably closer to the truth to think of stress as a trigger factor rather than a direct cause.

Having run through the suspects list – and, who knows, the vital mystery factor X causing breast cancer may yet be awaiting discovery – this is the moment to clear up a few misconceptions which can cause women needless worry and unhappiness. A knock, a blow or a fall does *not* cause breast cancer. It is not infectious, it is not unclean and it is not, strictly speaking, hereditary except in the rather remote sense that a daughter may inherit some of her mother's predisposing genetic characteristics.

Although so much is still unknown about breast cancer, we should not take the attitude that we are completely helpless to combat it. In the next chapter we shall be looking at some of the positive things we can do to reduce our risk.

[3]

What are we looking for?

Breast cancer is not preventable, as yet. Even when the medical scientists do find answers to the many questions they are asking about causes, the solutions may still not be readily apparent. This currently leaves us only two ways in which we can hope to improve the cure rates for this form of cancer. The first is earlier detection. The second is finding better methods of treatment.

Early detection is important because the smaller the tumour the greater the likelihood that it will not have spread into the lymph nodes and the better, therefore, the chances of cure. It also usually means that less drastic treatment can be offered. However, the size of the tumour, although significant for the doctor when making a diagnosis, is not an invariable indicator for making a prognosis because there are twenty or more pathological types of breast cancer and some are more aggressive than others; in plain words, they grow faster and spread more rapidly.

The type of cancer and the stage it has reached will influence the doctor's thinking about treatment. There are now many variations and combinations available and although no therapy can promise certain cure, there is definitely more cause for optimism. Some of the treatments appear to be achieving improved outcomes when measured in terms of longer survival and periods of time free from cancer. More certainty about the long-term effects of treatment has also made it possible for doctors to offer more women less disfiguring surgery. The details of these treatments are discussed in chapters 7 and 8.

EARLY DETECTION

How early is early? This is a problem which still baffles the oncologists, the people who specialise in cancer. Tumour cells grow by doubling. One cancer cell becomes two, then four, eight, sixteen, and so on. Some tumours grow rapidly, doubling themselves every few days; others take a year or more; but where it has been possible to measure them, it seems the average doubling rate is somewhere between one and five months. However, not all tumours follow the same pattern, so although, broadly speaking, a tiny tumour indicates early disease, and a large one indicates advanced disease, a disturbing number of early lesions which may show up on a mammogram as no more than a slight alteration in the tissue will prove, on further investigation, to be already invasive – that is to say, the cancer has spread to the lymph nodes.

The smallest tumour a mammogram can pick up is about half a centimetre in size; the smallest tumour a woman or her doctor can feel is about two centimetres. In fact, the average-size tumour that a woman will pick up through breast self-examination is three centimetres. Given that a centimetre of tumour represents one gram of tissue – which is about a billion cells, or thirty doubling times – and could have taken anything from three to eight years to grow in what is known as the 'silent interval', the nature of the problem becomes evident. It suggests that some seemingly 'early' breast cancers could have been present for many years.

This certainly does not mean that it is impossible to detect genuinely early breast tumours, but it does imply that it is not always quite as straightforward a matter as is often suggested. Meanwhile, until we know how to prevent breast cancer, detection as early as we can achieve it, followed up by prompt remedial action, remain our best and main lines of defence.

So how do we do this detection? There are three methods: two are medical – clinical examination and mammography – and these depend on a woman presenting herself to a doctor, either for screening or because she is troubled by some symptoms in her breast. The third is breast self-examination, or BSE as it is usually called.

Of the two medical methods the most recent, mammography, is highly effective in that it is an X-ray technique which can discover tumours before they are either visible or palpable. However, it does not supersede the traditional clinical examination, which involves a careful manual and visual inspection of both breasts. This latter procedure, particularly when it is done by a skilled and experienced doctor, remains an indispensable part of diagnosis. Nowadays, the clinical examination will be done as a prelude to mammography and will sometimes even reveal a tumour which does not show up on the mammogram. BSE is the same kind of manual examination as a doctor does, but it is carried out by the woman herself.

BREAST AWARENESS

Although BSE has certain obvious limitations – for a start, the fact that it is done by a non-medical person and should never, therefore, be regarded as a complete alternative to either medical screening or diagnosis – it does also have some important advantages, particularly for the well woman, which make it a very useful back-up method for early detection.

In the first place it is something positive a woman can do for herself, in the privacy of her bedroom and at a convenient time. BSE is, quite literally, within her own hands to accomplish and this can only be good psychologically, both for her morale and for her sense of self-esteem. We simply cannot allow ourselves to rely entirely on doctors and the medical technology now available to them to maintain us in a good state of health. As far as possible we should seek to be in charge of our own bodies, so the more we know about sound preventive health measures, and act on them, the better able we will be to make the important decisions when the need arises.

Possibly the supreme advantages of breast self-examination is that it enables a woman to familiarise herself with the shape, feel and appearance of her breasts in a *normal* condition – this includes all the swellings, tenderness and other changes that many women habitually experience in the course of their monthly cycle. In a more subtle way, it helps her to overcome any lingering inhibitions she may have about her body generally, so that should she find it necessary to visit her doctor because she thinks there may be something wrong with any part of her, she will feel less reluctant about discussing her problem. (As we shall see later on in this book, sensitive, open communication between doctor and patient is vital for a relationship which has trust as its cornerstone and cannot thrive without it.)

Most adolescent girls are keenly interested in the development of their breasts and they may spend long hours gazing at themselves in the mirror, probably agonising unnecessarily because they don't measure up to some impossible ideal. They worry that their breasts are the wrong size, the wrong shape or embarrassingly protuberant; they may resent them because they hinder their sporting activities or feel ashamed of them because they draw unwanted attention from boys. Whether they welcome them or dread them, girls at this age are acutely aware of these unequivocal signals that they are entering womanhood.

This heightened perception at the beginning of conscious sexuality sometimes becomes curiously introverted or denied as women become older, particularly after the menopause, when they may think or perhaps are made to feel that an active sexual life is over for them. Many older women seem almost afraid to look at their breasts, let alone touch them. If this is a problem for you, don't be ashamed of it. We are not all made the same, psychologically any more than physically, and some people are naturally more modest about their bodies or may find it more difficult to overcome the effects of an upbringing which, by today's standards, may have been strict or prudish. For the sake of your own health, however, it is important to try and cope with these inhibitions. The guidance on how to do breast self-examination includes suggestions for ways of breaking yourself in gently to the idea.

There is another reason why many women are turned off the idea of breast self-examination. It is not that they don't know that they should report anything unusual like a lump or a discharge; quite the contrary, they know full well what they should do, but they also believe they can predict what the doctor's verdict will be, and they don't want to hear it. In most women's minds breast lumps are automatically associated with breast cancer, and that can mean only two things: losing their breast and possibly their life. With this negative outlook – shared, unfortunately, by some health professionals – it is hardly surprising that many women are reluctant to take even the first precautionary steps of doing self-examination.

Here are some positive scientific facts to counter these understandable fears. *Nine out of ten lumps are benign* – that is to say, no cancer is present. If you are under thirty the probability that the lump is harmless is even higher. (Only one per cent of all breast cancers occur in women in the youngest age groups). All the same, and whatever your age, any abnormality should always be reported, if only to put your mind at rest.

Another fact: the sooner the lump is found *and medically investigated*, the better your chances for cure. Furthermore, the treatment available for a breast cancer which has been presented to a doctor immediately on discovery is likely to be less radical and disfiguring than if the delay has reached the point where a mastectomy is the only solution or, worse still, the cancer may have become inoperable.

Another unenviable British record is that in this country 20 per cent of women present with inoperable advanced cancer compared to only 10 per cent in the other European countries. Many of these women are elderly and single, which may partially explain why they have not visited the doctor earlier, and this is the group where the disease is most prevalent; yet it could be treated reasonably conservatively if it were diagnosed early enough. So if you have a mother or aunt or maybe older friends whom you suspect may be taking an ostrich-like attitude to their health, do try to persuade them of the value of regular BSE. You could set them a good example by showing them how to do it.

Many women have naturally lumpy breasts. Others suffer from benign disease of one sort or another which may fluctuate with the menstrual cycle, making the breasts swollen and painful at certain times in the month, usually just before the period. It is also quite usual for breasts to look slightly different. For instance, one may be larger or set lower than the other. Breasts also change internally as the woman grows older. From being dense, glandular structures admirably suited for their prime function of suckling a baby, they gradually become less glandular and more fatty until in a woman's later years, after the menopause, fat has almost entirely replaced the glandular tissue. Eventually the fat too reduces, giving the breasts a characteristically shrunken (atrophic) appearance in old age.

The woman who has trained herself to feel her breasts regularly and knows about these normal changes will not be alarmed by them; at the same time, just because she knows her breasts so well, she will also know how to pick up an unexpected change. This is yet another very important advantage of breast self-examination. The woman who knows her own breasts well can often sense intuitively, even before feeling anything tangible, when something may be going wrong. One very experienced surgeon, who examines on average two thousand breasts a year, told me that he still sometimes finds himself searching for a lump, but if the patient is a woman who is familiar with breast self-examination, she can often pinpoint it accurately for him. She, after all, lives with her breasts and is therefore likely to be the first to be aware of any changes.

BREAST SELF-EXAMINATION – HOW TO DO IT

Although 90 per cent of breast cancers present as a lump, there are other warning signs for which a woman should be on the alert when she does her monthly examination. Basically, you are looking for abnormal change, any alteration in the shape, look or feel of your breasts which you know is not part of your monthly cycle. Maybe you think you already know what these changes are, but just in case you forget or miss one out, why not copy out this list and slip it into the corner of the mirror when you do your examination?

Breast   Change in shape

Change in size (usually larger but sometimes appears to be shrinking; feels harder)

Change in skin texture – a rash, puckering or dimpling

Enlarged veins

Lump or thickening anywhere

A persistently painful area in either breast which feels different from pre-menstrual tenderness

Nipple   Discharge (any colour, any consistency)

Retraction (drawing in)

Rash on nipple or areola (brown skin surrounding the nipple)

Lump or thickening round or under it

Change in texture

Arm   Swelling of upper arm

Swelling in the armpit or above the breast (enlarged lymph or pectoral nodes)

The three Rs

Breast self-examination is neither difficult nor complicated once you have mastered the order of action, but if it is to be any real use it does require the following three Rs from you: Regularity, Relaxation and Repetition.

Regularity means choosing a day of the month and always doing it on that day, no matter what else may be crowded into it. Pre-menopausal women are advised to do it immediately after their period ends, when their breasts are likely to be at their softest and least lumpy. Women after the menopause can pick any day of the month – for example, always the first or the last – to help them to remember it.

Relaxation means giving yourself the peace and privacy you need to carry out this examination in a concentrated, careful and unhurried way. For those women who may find it a strange procedure at first – and it does take getting used to – doing it in the bath is a good way to start. To wash properly you have to touch your body all over anyway. When it is time to examine your breasts, drop your flannel or sponge and run your soapy hands round, over and under them. This is a good way of feeling for lumps, and it will help you to feel less nervous and tense next time. The whole examination takes between five and ten minutes and you do not want to be interrupted in the middle of it because you might miss out a stage, so if there are people in the house who could disturb you, lock the door.

Repetition means doing exactly the same routine in the same order every time. Here it is:

LOOKING (INVESTIGATING)

1. Strip to the waist. Sit or stand in front of a mirror with a good light, your arms hanging loosely by your sides, and look at your breasts carefully, noting their shape, their size and whether they differ in any way from each other. It is quite normal for breasts and nipples to be asymmetrical but it is important for you to be aware of that image, looking at yourself the same way next time and every time thereafter so that you can be sure of spotting a change should one appear.

2. Slowly swing your arms up above your head, watching your breasts lift. Keeping your arms straight above your head, clasp your hands and press them forwards. Continue to gaze at your reflection very carefully, looking for any distortion or change in the outline of your breasts. Then look downwards at your nipples, checking for any unusual change in their position or appearance.

3. Slowly swing your arms down and forwards, keeping them level with your shoulders and your hands clasped. Look at your nipples as they move, again checking for any unusual change.

4. Place your hands on your hips and press firmly downwards and inwards until you feel your chest muscles tighten. Look for any unusual change in skin texture (puckering or dimpling) or nipple retraction. Lean forwards so that your breasts hang free from your ribcage. Check again for changes in outline or skin texture.

5. Look at the underside of your breasts to check for unusual reddening or other changes.

6. Examine the inside of your bra for blood or any other non-milky discharge.

FEELING (PALPATION)

Lie on your bed in a relaxed position, a low pillow under your head and a folded towel under the shoulder on the side that is to be examined. Examine each breast in turn: left breast with right hand and right breast with left hand.

1. *Left breast*: Start with your left arm under your head. Using your right hand and with fingers flat and close together, press the pads of your fingers in small circular movements all round the breast. Start centrally above the nipple and move firmly but gently round your breast – outwards, downwards, inwards and upwards. Continue pressing spirally until you have covered the whole surface of your breast – at least two circles and probably more, depending on the size of your breast.

2. Keeping fingers flat, move up to the collarbone and across to the centre of your chest.

3. Bring your left arm down beside you, and with the fingers of your right hand firmly press the side of your left breast and into your left armpit with the circular motion described above.

4. *Right breast*: Put the towel under your right shoulder; reverse and repeat the procedure.

If you prefer, you can do the palpation bit of breast self-examination in the bath or under the shower, using your soapy fingers.

Once you have been through this exercise two or three times, you will wonder why you ever worried about it. Try not to become anxious about getting it exactly right. It is much more important to be doing something rather than nothing, and practice will soon make you adequately proficient.

There are many illustrated leaflets available which give you a step-by-step guide to BSE; the addresses of the organisations supplying them are listed in Resources. There are also some good videos which can be bought or hired, but you do need to see them at least twice to memorise them accurately. If you belong to a women's organisation or a trade union, or work for a company with a declared interest in promoting the health of its employees, it might be worth suggesting that such a video be hired and shown at a time when the maximum number of women can attend.

There is absolutely no need to do BSE more than once a month. Once you have finished your self-examination, and providing you have found no change, you can forget about your breasts until the same time next month.

But what if you do find something unusual? You must, without delay, make an appointment to see your doctor. Do not, in the interval, press the lump or squeeze the nipple. Whatever it is, leave it alone but remember, *nine out of ten lumps are benign.*

[4]

I've got a lump in my breast

DON'T DELAY!

Before the advent of screening about 95 per cent of breast lumps were found by the woman herself, or by her partner. Even when the national breast screening progamme is in full operation – and that will take a few years to achieve – most lumps and other suspicious breast symptoms will continue to be discovered by women themselves, irrespective of whether they do regular breast self-examination. Approximately 80 per cent of women are well aware that they should tell their doctor about a lump in their breast, but not so many know that other changes (described in chapter 3) should also be reported. Some 25 per cent of women who do find an abnormality delay three months or longer before taking themselves to the docor's surgery.

Why do they do this? Research studies have shown that it is unlikely to be due to complete ignorance. A survey of patients at a Southampton hospital showed that older women delayed longer than younger women, and patients with benign disease reported more swiftly than those who were ultimately diagnosed with breast cancer.[1] This suggests first, that younger women are more likely to know – and more importantly, believe that early detection gives them an improved chance of cure – and second, that women are their own best judges of knowing when something is wrong with their health. The women who correctly guessed that they did have cancer were understandably reluctant to have their worst fears confirmed. An interesting but somewhat depressing follow-up to this survey is that despite a health education campaign in the area, which was directed at GPs as well as women, the delay figures did not improve.

Clearly, being informed and knowing what you ought to do is not enough. People must be convinced that there is a positive benefit for them before they will be ready to act on that knowledge. Fear is a more likely reason for delay: fear, first of all, that it will prove to be cancer, a word which spells death to most people; and second, fear of losing a breast which, for some women, can be an even more potent cause for delay. Most of us share these fears, so what is the extra factor which makes one in four women delay so dangerously?

It appears that age, class, education, marital status, pain or its absence, and many other indicators which psychologists use for measurement purposes have little or no bearing on women's behaviour in this situation. When fear is acute – as it is, for instance, of a diagnosis of cancer – one way of dealing with the fear – and this is quite a common reaction – is to try to deny it. The calm woman who measures low levels of anxiety on the psychologist's questionnaire may in reality be suppressing terrifying emotions, a sense of helplessness in the face of overwhelming panic or feelings of isolation and abandonment. Denial may be characteristic of the way she deals with other difficult or stressful situations in her life, so to those who do not know her well she may appear admirably in control. A serene, apparently unruffled demeanour in the midst of crises which would reduce other people to tears or rage or shivering apprehension can be deceptive. Only she knows what a quivering jelly she is inside but, if she plays the game successfully for long enough, she may end up convincing herself that there is nothing to worry about.

Thus when she feels a lump, she will immediately reassure herself – 'It can't be serious' or 'It can't happen to me' – and try to shut it out of her mind. Many such women will probably not even open this book when they see what it is about, dismissing it as 'morbid curiosity' or 'getting all steamed up about something which may never happen'. Of course we all hope it won't, but hoping for the best is not a reason for avoiding knowledge of the facts. There is sound sense in the old adage which says that to be forewarned is to be forearmed.

It is so easy to find 'good' reasons for avoiding something unpleasant: being too busy, waiting until after the long-planned family holiday, or convincing yourself that you are making a fuss about nothing. Fear can make cowards or fools of us all, and we do not always react instinctively in our own best interests. So while it is perfectly understandable to fear cancer, we must try not to let our apprehension cause us to lose balance or make us obsessively anxious.

Cancer phobia is very distressing for those who suffer from it, and it is the reverse of suppressing anxiety. In these cases fear becomes unbridled and all-absorbing. The most ordinary physical symptom immediately assumes a sinister implication, and this may lead to having extended and unnecessary clinical tests. Very often the phobia has been triggered by some quite different psychological problem which needs to be recognised before it can be treated appropriately.

Although it is important not to be overanxious, it is equally unwise to take a fatalistic 'What will be will be' kind of attitude. So many people believe that if they are 'doomed' to get cancer there is nothing they can do about it, and that no treatment can affect the final bound-to-be-fatal outcome.

This is just not true. Cancer is curable. In Britain alone, it is estimated that some 75,000 people are cured of cancer *every year*, many of them women with breast or cervical cancer, because these are both conditions with a good prognosis if they are found really early.

TALKING TO YOUR DOCTOR

Anything slightly unusual in the appearance of your breasts must be reported immediately to your GP. Don't be afraid of what he or she may say, or that you will be laughed at for being foolishly overanxious. Most family doctors are sensible, sympathetic people who take their patients' worries seriously, but you cannot expect them to have telepathic powers. If you do not explain what is wrong with you, the doctor is not going to be able to guess unless he or she happens to be an exceptionally sensitive and experienced person who can pick up anxiety vibes from across the desk.

Many women who are worried about their health find it hard, once they are actually in the doctor's surgery, to admit their anxiety. If the doctor is a man, the woman patient may feel embarrassed about explaining a symptom like a breast lump or vaginal discharge which will involve her having an intimate examination, so she may produce some trivial complaint in another part of her body, like a sore throat, or use her child's health as an excuse for coming to see him.

Most experienced doctors are aware of these avoidance tactics and will make it a routine part of their practice to enquire about their patient's general health. If they have not seen her for some time they ought to check to see whether she has had her cervical smear test; they should ask whether she has had any unusual pain or discharge in her genital area; they should also suggest that they do a clinical breast examination and, if she is over fifty, recommend that she attend her local screening clinic. (See chapter 5 for more information on the national breast screening programme.) This is ideal medical practice, but do not rely on automatically receiving it.

You too are responsible for your own health, so if there is something which is seriously bothering you, screw up your courage, rub out your inhibitions and do not hesitate to make an appointment with the doctor *as soon as possible*. Once in his or her surgery, try to explain in as direct and exact a way as you can what is troubling you. If you feel very unnerved by the prospect, take your partner, a close relative or a friend with you. Even if they do not go beyond the waiting room, their very presence outside and the knowledge that you could call them in if you needed to will give you strength and support.

Unfortunately, just as there are some doctors who will do everything to help their patients through a difficult examination, there is a minority which is too apathetic, too 'busy' or too intolerant to pay proper attention to patients unless they are almost dead on their feet. There are also a few male doctors who are always going to be somewhat defensive or aloof towards their female patients, perhaps because they do not like women very much or are afraid that they may be accused of improper behaviour. This is obviously a rare attitude, particularly nowadays when there are so many large group practices with usually a nurse in attendance, but it is worth remembering that doctors have personal problems like the rest of us, and may be no better at dealing with them.

The doctor to beware of is the one who looks at your lump, or whatever other symptom it may be, usually somewhat perfunctorily, and then says, 'Nothing to worry about! Come back in a month [or six months] if it is still there.' Even though it may mean an unpleasant few minutes, refuse to take this for an answer and *never* wait to see what happens. Although it is hard for patients to stand up to their doctors and demand a second opinion, in a situation like this you can be sure that such an answer is never satisfactory.

Any abnormal change in the breast should always be submitted to further examination. One breast specialist goes so far as to say that in his opinion, if a woman is worried about the possibility of breast cancer, even without any apparent symptoms, that is a medical symptom in itself and justifies the GP referring her to a fully equipped breast unit where she can have a complete examination.

AT THE BREAST CLINIC

Family doctors will see only a very few suspicious breast symptoms during a year's practice and they are, therefore, not likely to be very skilled at palpating breasts unless they have made a point of doing this as part of their routine examination of women patients. Nor are they in a position to make a firm diagnosis of cancer because this requires technology which is available only in hospitals. The best the GP can do is to make an intelligent guess about the nature of the symptom. The conscientious GP will, therefore, if he or she finds anything abnormal, however slight, recommend a woman to see a consultant, on the grounds that it is better to be safe than sorry.

This must be your attitude too. Furthermore, it is most important that you be referred to a breast specialist who is backed up by all the facilities of a well-equipped breast unit and a multidisciplinary medical team. Since cancer of the breast is a relatively common disease, there are too many general surgeons about who reckon that they know how to deal with it – just a simple matter of cut and remove. However, unless they have developed a particular interest in breast surgery, they probably do no more than a dozen breast operations a year, if that, and these will invariably be mastectomies. This does not qualify them as specialists in a disease which anyway, as we shall see later, cannot be treated adequately with surgery alone.

One of the good fall-out aspects of the newly launched national breast screening programme is that there will soon be many more breast clinics around the country to which symptomatic women of any age can be referred and where they will be certain of receiving attention from breast specialists. With slight variations in procedure, this is what you can expect to happen at a well-run clinic when you go for your first appointment.

The doctor starts by taking a *medical history* which will pay particular attention to hormonal factors (your menstrual pattern, number of pregnancies, dates of menarche, menopause, and so on), your family background (is there a history of breast cancer?) and any previous breast problems you may have had.

This is followed by a *clinical examination* in which the

doctor begins by making a visual inspection of the symptomatic breast, comparing its appearance with the other one. Then, with the woman in both sitting and lying positions, he carefully palpates the breast, much in the manner that was described in the previous chapter for breast self-examination. The general appearance of the breast is very significant to the experienced clinician. If you have spotted any of those warning signs on your list, the doctor will see them too and will want to know when you first noticed them. If you have delayed reporting them, do not make things worse now by pretending that you have only just discovered them. It is crucially important for the consultant to have all the facts in order to make the correct diagnosis, so do answer all questions truthfully.

After the doctor has examined the symptomatic breast and felt carefully in the armpit and at the base of the neck for enlarged lymph nodes, he or she will examine the other breast with equal thoroughness. By this time the doctor will have a fairly good idea of the nature of the problem: whether it is some form of benign disease – which will be the case nine times out of ten – or whether it could possibly be a malignancy. Some cancers are immediately obvious to the experienced doctor. Unhappily, this is often because the woman has delayed until it has progressed to a stage where it is visibly diagnosable. However, sometimes it is because of the type of cancer she has – either very fast-growing or highly inflamed.

The doctor no longer relies on a clinical judgement alone for a diagnosis, so your clinical examination will now be followed by a visit to the radiology department, where you will have a mammogram.

Mammography is an X-ray technique which has been specially developed for taking pictures of soft fatty tissue. The larger and, therefore, the more fatty the breast, the better the picture that will be produced, because any lesions in the breast show up vividly against the fat. Conversely, mammography is less effective for women with small breasts which contain little fat and are probably much denser structures.

Although mammography can pick up very minor pre-cancerous changes, called microcalcifications, it can also sometimes miss lumps which have been felt in the clinical examination (about 5 per cent). This fact underlines the importance of always combining mammography with a clinical examination, and it is invariably used for assessing symptomatic women over thirty-five, irrespective of whether there are clinical signs of abnormality.

Mammographic techniques are improving all the time and the radiation dose has been steadily reduced until today the risk of a mammogram causing cancer has been described as roughly equivalent to smoking a third of a cigarette once a year. However, it should always be used with care. Whatever a woman's age – and the older she is, the less risk she runs – she should not have a mammogram more frequently than once a year. Generally speaking, it is inadvisable for a woman under the age of thirty to have a mammogram unless the doctor has strong clinical reasons to believe that there is a suspicious abnormality which needs more precise localisation.

Mammography is also useful for detecting previously unsuspected abnormalities in another part of the breast or in the opposite one. In effect, it serves as a double check on the doctor's clinical examination which may inadvertently have tended to concentrate on the symptomatic breast. Surveys have shown that the average pick-up rate for an accurate diagnosis of cancer is between 85 and 90 per cent when it is done by a radiologist reading a mammogram. When surgeon and radiologist work together, their combined accuracy achieves 98 per cent, each picking up a few different cases; the one or two which remain to be detected may be missed out altogether or may have been diagnosed as benign (false negative) but on biopsy turn out to be malignant. False positives – lesions which are suspected to be malign but on further investigation prove to be non-cancerous – are discussed in chapter 5.

Ultrasound is sometimes used to complement the mammogram, usually to assist in determining the nature of the lump. If it is solid it will probably require an excision biopsy (see below) but if it is a cyst then all that may be necessary is to draw off the fluid with a fine needle.

There are also a few enthusiasts who persist with *thermography* because they believe it has a special role to play in diagnosing breast cancer. It is a completely harmless means of measuring, by infra-red radiation, the varying heat patterns of the body. About 85 per cent of cancers are hot, and the degree of heat tends to be a prognostic indicator in itself. The breasts are first cooled; then any 'hot spot' which is picked up indicates an abnormality, but this may not necessarily be a malignancy. And herein lies a major problem with thermograms: they pick up a lot of 'false positives' which, on further examination, prove non-cancerous. Equally, they can pick up 'false negatives' which would be even more dangerous if they were not counter-checked by a mammogram.

If the doctor thinks you have a cyst – very common in women between thirty-five and fifty-five, and usually very recognisable because it tends to be mobile and feel soft and springy to the touch, rather like a tiny balloon – he or she will draw off the liquid there and then. *Fine-needle aspiration cytology*, as it is called, is a quick, virtually painless procedure requiring no anaesthetic. It is the reverse of an injection: the doctor inserts a very fine needle into the head of the cyst and aspirates all the fluid, which may be yellow or dark in colour, into a syringe. The cyst is deflated and nothing further need be done unless there are signs of blood in the fluid, in which case it may be necessary to do a biopsy. Some doctors always have the cystic fluid analysed just to be on the safe side. No one is sure why cysts happen – too much coffee-drinking has been suggested as one cause, but it is unproven. Although cysts are harmless, they are tiresome and worrying until they have been treated. They also have a way of recurring time after time, and they should always be seen by a doctor.

This same process of fine-needle aspiration cytology can also be used for diagnosing solid lumps. The doctor draws out a tiny sample of tissue containing a cluster of cells from the centre of the lump and sends it immediately to the laboratory for analysis. This is a very accurate and swift diagnostic method, providing that both clinician and cytologist are experienced – one more good reason for consulting a surgeon with a special interest in breast cancer.

Should the lump be very large or if there is not a good cytology service to interpret the results of fine-needle aspiration, the doctor may prefer to do what is called a *tru-cut* or *drill biopsy*. The area of the lump is defined, local anaesthetic is infiltrated through the skin, a needle larger than that used in the aspiration procedure described above is inserted, and with it the doctor cuts out a small core of tissue. This too is sent to the laboratory, where it will go through all the necessary histological tests to determine the nature of the tumour. The results will not come through immediately, which means having to return to the clinic, or wait by the telephone, for a few days. If the results are positive the surgeon knows definitely that cancer is present, but if they are negative they cannot be accepted at face value. The whole lump has to be removed in a small operation under a general anaesthetic and sent back to the laboratory for a repeat analysis.

This procedure is called an *open (excision) biopsy* and it is done in all cases where a cancer is suspected, but a definite diagnosis cannot be obtained in any other way.

The development of safe aspiration procedures which can be done on the spot and without general anaesthetic, coupled with the high degree of accuracy now possible through mammographic diagnosis, has meant that many women can be spared the anguish of surgery for what will turn out to be a benign condition. It is worth emphasising that most women who have arrived in the breast clinic because they have symptoms will leave it reassured that there is nothing seriously wrong with them.

BAD NEWS

One in five women will not be so lucky. Either their cancer will have been diagnosed at this first visit, or they will have to go into hospital for an excision biopsy and further investigation. If cancer is definitely present, they will need to undergo further tests to see whether the cancer has spread (metastasised) to other parts of the body. The most usual sites for secondary breast cancer are in the bones, the lungs, the liver and sometimes the brain. Scans will be done of all these organs as part of the process of diagnosing the clinical stage of the disease, whether or not the woman has symptoms, and usually she will not. (See chapter 6 for more information about the criteria for the clinical staging of tumours.)

From the doctor's point of view, the ability to diagnose cancer through fine-needle aspiration cytology has the great merit of saving time and being cost-effective because if cancer is established (it provides a definite diagnosis in 85 per cent of cancers presenting as a solid lump), the woman can be informed there and then. During the same visit she can be sent for further tests to check for spread of cancer, and her treatment plan can be drawn up and discussed with her.

From the woman's point of view, both the diagnosis and this swift processing through the various ensuing tests are likely to cause her great distress. She may not have been at all prepared psychologically for a bad diagnosis, so if the doctor has a brusque manner or she is unaccompanied by a husband or relative and the nurses are scurrying around, clearly too preoccupied to give her time to unburden herself — all quite possible scenarios in today's busy NHS outpatient departments — she may leave the hospital devastated and desperate.

It is hard to say whether it is worse to receive bad news when you are not ready for it, or after you have endured a week or more of waiting and hoping against hope. Probably the latter situation is more bearable because at least you will have had time to talk it over with someone close to you. Much, of course, depends on the way the information is disclosed, and this is largely the responsibility of the consultant and the nurses. One thing is absolutely certain: no one who has just been told they have cancer should ever be allowed to leave an outpatient clinic on their own, yet sadly this happens far too often. Kind, sensitive communication is an essential part of the good treatment and care of cancer patients. We shall return to this subject in later chapters.

[5]

Screening could save your life

A few years ago this chapter title would have been unthinkable. Rightly, it would have been regarded as a grossly irresponsible statement, raising expectations that had no hope of being met. But recently the whole picture has been transformed from grey uncertainty to a sunnier landscape of reasonably founded optimism, at least for women over the age of fifty. What has caused this shift of opinion? How is it justified? Why is there an age bar?

SCREENING TRIALS

To answer these questions we need to go back to the mid sixties when the first long-term, large-scale trial of breast cancer screening was set up in the United States for women members of the Health Insurance Plan (HIP) of New York. (HIP, rather like BUPA or PPP in this country, is a private medical insurance scheme.)

Between 1963 and 1969, 62,000 women between forty and sixty-four, all living within the greater New York area, were randomly allocated to one of two groups: 31,000 to the study group who were offered screening for breast cancer and the other 31,000 to the control group who did not receive any more than the usual medical care. In other words, this latter group were not given mammograms, neither did they undergo other investigations unless they presented themselves with symptoms, whereas the screening group received an initial examination which included taking a detailed medical, social and family history, followed by a clinical examination, mammography and thermography. The screened women were then asked to return for three further annual check-ups.

Even though 10,000 women refused the invitation to participate in the study group (one-third) and despite, too, the inevitable disappearance of women from HIP records after five years (about 20 per cent in both groups) careful follow-up, now approaching twenty years, shows a consistent *one-third reduction in the number of deaths from breast cancer among women over fifty in the study group*. There has also been some decline in the number of deaths for younger women, those between forty and forty-nine, but not enough to be significant in statistical terms.

Following the HIP interim report, which published its first encouraging figures five years after the women's entry to the screening programme, other countries decided to set up their own trials. Between 1977 and 1984 Sweden offered screening on a randomly allocated basis (half and half) to nearly 135,000 women between forty and seventy-four. Those in the study group were offered screening by mammography alone, every two or three years, the length of this interval depending on their age. The acceptance rate was very high – 89 per cent of the women invited agreed to participate – and by the end of 1984 the results matched the American ones. Overall, 31 per cent fewer women in the study group had died from breast cancer but again, as with the American trial, there was no significant decline in mortality for the younger women, between forty and forty-nine, although there was some improvement.

Two distinct trials in Holland also started in the mid seventies using different designs – one with mammography alone, the other combining it with a clinical examination – but both yielded the same main conclusion: that women in the fifty-plus age group who accepted screening for breast cancer reduced their relative risk of dying from the disease by half. In both towns (Utrecht and Nijmegen), involving 43,000 women in all, the acceptance rates were high: 72 per cent and 85 per cent respectively.

The largest screening trial of all, in the sense of numbers of women participating (240,000) and centres (eight), was started in the United Kingdom in 1979. It was planned to last seven years, and its aim was to assess the relative merits of two screening programmes, designed differently but both using mammography and clinical examination (at Edinburgh and Guildford), and to compare them with breast self-examination programmes, also taught and run along different lines (at Huddersfield and Nottingham). The other four control centres (Dundee, Oxford, Southmead and Stoke-on-Trent) were used for comparison and were matched as closely as possible for demographic features such as class, proportion of urban to rural inhabitants, and spread of occupations. A similar group of women between forty-five and sixty-four in these control centres was identified but not contacted.

The first results on mortality in the UK trial were published in *The Lancet* in August 1988[1] and although they are not as good as the Swedish or American figures – over the first five years there is only a 20 per cent reduction in deaths for screened women – this still counts as a significant improvement. The authors of the paper, who are also the co-ordinators of the trial, offer three suggestions to explain these less good results: the mammographic techniques may not have been as refined; many women did not receive their screening invitations because of inadequate GP registers; and finally, among those who did, the acceptance rate was markedly lower than in either Sweden or Holland (60 per cent in Edinburgh and 72 per cent in Guildford the first time and reducing slightly with each screening round).

This last factor may say something about our culture or our level of health awareness, or both, but whatever it is, any screening programme is doomed to expensive failure if not enough of the targeted population takes advantage of it. Even before these results were published, the government had already announced its intention of setting up a national screening programme for women between fifty and sixty-four. This decision was based on the recommendations of the Forrest Report (the title taken from Professor Sir Patrick Forrest, the chairman of the working party set up in 1985 to investigate the pros and cons for such a programme).[2] There are cynics who would say that this decision, so triumphantly announced on the day the Forrest Report was published and only a few weeks before the general election in June 1986, evinced as much a concern for political expediency as for women's health, but does this matter if ultimately the right outcome is achieved?

THE NATIONAL BREAST SCREENING PROGRAMME

The first centres were opened in April 1987 and by 1990 the Department of Health intends to have established 100 screening centres throughout the country, including mobile units for rural areas. Each centre will serve a population of about half a million. At least £55 million has been earmarked for getting this programme fully on the road and this includes costs for staff training, computer software (to analyse results and operate the call and recall system, among other things) and health education.

All women between fifty and sixty-four are eligible to enter the programme which entitles them to a mammogram at three-yearly intervals. They will be invited through their GPs and their names will be registered so that they can be recalled on the appropriate date. If you are in this age group but for some reason you have not heard of this programme nor yet received an invitation from your family doctor – perhaps you have changed address or moved to another district and not registered with a new GP – it is not too late to take advantage of it. Simply ask your doctor to make an appointment for you.

Women over sixty-five can ask to be screened if they wish,

and no doubt those who have been through the programme will want to continue. Younger women are not eligible because up to now mammography has not proved very good at detecting their early cancers, particularly in those under forty. This is mainly because the denser structure of the breast makes the picture harder to interpret, but there is also the matter of hard economics, which cannot be ignored. It is simply not cost-effective to screen a large population in which relatively few cancers occur.

However, as both the technology and the expertise to operate it improve, this may change. The age factor is being kept under review – should it be lowered to forty-five? – as is the length of screening intervals – should they be brought down to two years or even one? Other areas of continuing research include monitoring the way further investigations are carried out and whether women who do need further investigation become unduly anxious.

This programme is an expensive and ambitious initative and one that has no model elsewhere, so for once this country can justifiably claim credit for taking the lead in an important area of health care. However, even some of the more enthusiastic proponents of screening are preaching caution on several counts. They are particularly concerned about the current shortage of suitably trained personnel, especially radiographers and radiologists, but this is a problem with a finite solution – provided, of course, that the government makes sufficient money available. More imponderable, and a question which will take longer to resolve, is how women will respond to screening and whether they fully appreciate what it can and cannot offer them.

Dr Petr Skrabanek, a lecturer in community health at the University of Dublin, is a critic who is positively against screening and manages to produce figures which contradict all the accepted results from the trials. Arguing about statistics is one thing, and we probably all agree with Mark Twain that they can be used to say almost anything, including falsehoods. The real trouble with statistics is that they refer to an abstract entity – a population – whereas what we worry about as individuals is what screening can do for us – or not, as the case may be. So is Skrabanek correct when he accuses the Forrest working party (of which he was a dissenting member) and the Department of Health of offering false promises based on false premises?[3]

He suggests, for example, that women are not being properly informed about the inherent limitations of breast cancer screening. Do they properly understand, for instance, that breast screening cannot prevent cancer in the way that cervical screening does, nor does 'early' detection automatically guarantee cure, for reasons already explained in chapter 3. Even if you do realise that a screen does not prevent breast cancer, it is important also to appreciate that an all-clear on a given day does not mean immunity and protection for ever after. Inevitably, some women are in for a nasty surprise when they go in for a routine screen, expecting to be cleared as usual, only to be told that this time the news is not good. And though early detection does give you a much higher chance of cure, there are always going to be some unlucky women who will not have such a good prognosis. In these cases, there is an argument that so-called early detection has merely given them bad news before they would normally have known it.

Another cause for Skrabanek's concern – and many doctors share it – is that there will be a large number of healthy women (one in ten) who will be put through further tests because their mammogram has shown up an abnormality which must be analysed. These further investigations may include surgery – an excision biopsy – and they will certainly cause considerable anxiety.

A screening programme is a preventative health measure imposed on a healthy population. Skrabanek believes that doctors have no right to offer a benefit to such a population, especially when it is of so slender a nature – no news is good news – unless this same population is also informed of the risks. False positives involving further investigations are bad enough; even more worrying is the possibility of a false reassurance bestowed by a false negative, which is what happens when the mammogram fails to detect a malignancy. To counter some of these problems he would like to see ethical guidelines drawn up for obtaining consent to screening, along the lines of those already existing for clinical research. For somewhat different reasons the medical defence unions are muttering the same thing, and it is easy to see why they should be concerned. An aggrieved woman who discovers that her lump was missed at screening might well want to sue.

A recently published guide for GPs asserts that 'breast cancer screening is offered to a woman with an explicit promise that it will do her some good and an implicit understanding that it will cause her no harm.'[4] The best way we can judge for ourselves the merits of breast cancer screening is to follow the experts on the Forrest working party: they measured present facilities for detecting and treating early breast cancer against certain widely accepted principles for screening.

PRINCIPLES OF SCREENING APPLIED TO BREAST CANCER[5]

1 *The condition to be screened for poses an important health problem.* Yes.

2 *The natural history of the disease should be well understood.* It is not.

3 *There should be a recognisable early stage.* In the case of breast cancer this means disease which has not spread beyond the breast. It is estimated that about 45 per cent of the cancers detected by mammography at the first screen are small enough to be described as early stage.

4 *Treatment of the disease at an early stage should be of more benefit than treatment started at a later stage.* Despite

the variability of breast cancer, it is generally accepted that Stage I and Stage II cancers (see chapter 6) have a better prognosis, and it is not being unduly optimistic to predict a good outcome for about 70 to 80 per cent of screen-detected cancers.

5 *There should be a suitable test or examination.* Mammography is the only technique able to detect breast cancer at a very early stage. Its suitability is defined by its accuracy: that is to say, how *sensitive* is it − few false negatives − and how *specific* it is − few false positives. With screening intervals currently fixed at three years, it is estimated that between two and three women out of ten who have breast cancer may be missed at the screen. However, this may not be entirely due to lack of *sensitivity*, meaning that their cancer was missed by the mammogram (false negative); some fast-growing cancers will develop in the screening interval. As to *specificity*, with the current level of technology and expertise in using it, there will be about 10 per cent false positives. This means that one in ten screened women will have an 'abnormal' mammogram requiring further tests. The 'abnormality' usually means a technical problem about reading the mammogram and only two or three out of twenty of these so-called 'abnormal' mammograms will be serious possibilites for cancer. Of these, only one in twenty women will actually prove to have it.

6 *The test or examination should be acceptable to the population.* Experience from screening trials at Edinburgh and Guildford suggests that about 64 per cent of eligible women (two out of three) will respond to the first screening invitation and that numbers will gradually decline at subsequent screens. It appears that increasing age reduces the acceptability. The Forrest Report would like to see at least 70 per cent compliance, but even at the lower level a significant reduction in mortality can be achieved.

7 *There should be adequate available facilities for the diagnosis and treatment of detected abnormalities.* Women with

'abnormal' mammograms should be assessed without further delay, and this requires some or all of the investigations described in chapter 4. This means that there must be an assessment centre or breast clinic serviced by a multidisciplinary hospital team.

8 *For diseases of insidious onset, screening should be repeated at intervals determined by the natural history of the disease.* The optimum screening interval has yet to be determined but it is known that the incidence of cancer increases with age. The Swedish study concluded that annual screening would pick up 90 per cent of cancers present in those screened, biennial would pick up 80 per cent and triennial – the British choice – only 70 per cent. This decision is being kept under review.

9 *The chance of physical or psychological harm should be less than the chance of benefit.* Radiation risks are now very minimal, but there is the danger of 'over-diagnosis' and consequently over-investigation for very small lesions which may turn out to be harmless. Even if these tests cause little physical harm they may be psychologically distressing, regardless of whether the results turn out good or bad. The benefit is that a clear screen is reassuring, but it does not mean that a woman can relax her vigilance. This is where breast self-examination becomes very necessary to pick up any changes in the screening interval. The benefit of identifying a malignancy early will not be immediately obvious to a woman, but there is some comfort (and benefit) to be gained from the knowledge that she will need less radical treatment.

10 *The cost of a screening programme should be balanced against the benefit it provides.* The benefits for women are extra years of life and productivity, and less drastic treatment. The economic benefits, from the government's point of view, are the saving of productive lives and the saving in cost of treatment. How these costs are assessed and what is the real number of lives saved per year provides good fodder for

health economists, but the arguments are complex and difficult to follow for the lay person. Ultimately, the only realistic way to assess the success of the national breast screening programme will be to ask whether the number of lives it saves also saves money.

The Forrest Report has been criticised for being overoptimistic about compliance rates. A recent conservative evaluation[6] estimates that only about 8 per cent of lives could be saved, considerably less than the 30 per cent usually claimed. For England and Wales that amounts to 901 lives each year at a total cost per life saved of £39,000. The costs are estimated on the basis of combining the capital investment of setting up the programme with annual running costs. Although on this estimate the number of lives saved is far fewer than the 2,000 to 3,000 confidently claimed by many screening advocates, Professor George Knox, author of the paper, concedes that 'the attempt [to save lives by screening] is probably justified'.

As far as the individual post-menopausal woman is concerned, screening for breast cancer carries more pluses than minuses and she should take advantage of the programme, providing she is mentally prepared for all eventualities. It is not her problem to worry about whether the government can afford it.

WHAT HAPPENS AT THE SCREENING CENTRE

Screening for breast cancer is nothing like the embarrassing or painful ordeal many women fear. Procedures will obviously vary slightly from centre to centre but this is basically what to expect.

After giving the doctor or nurse a brief medical history, you will be taken to the radiography unit for the mammogram. Here you will be asked to strip to the waist, so it is sensible to wear a top of some kind with skirt or trousers rather than a dress. The radiographer will place each of your breasts in turn between two plastic or metal plates, depending on the machine used, to flatten them as far as possible so that a good picture can be taken. The squeeze is a bit uncomfortable but it lasts only for a few seconds and you will not feel any after-effects when your breast is released from what Judith Chalmers has called the 'booby trap'.

Your visit will last about half an hour. The film is read by a consultant radiologist and your GP will let you know the results in about ten days. If the mammogram is normal, nothing further need be done and you simply return for a screen in three years' time. If there is a technical problem about the picture you will be asked to come back for another mammogram, and in most cases this second screen will clear up the problem.

Should there be some abnormality you will be asked to attend an assessment centre, probably the nearest hospital breast clinic, where you will go through some of the tests described in chapter 4. These tests – which include a clinical examination, another mammogram, and probably fine-needle aspiration cytology – are done to establish whether the lesion is benign. If the news is good nothing further need be done, though you may be asked to come back for screening at an earlier interval just to keep an eye on things. If the lesion, however tiny and impalpable, still looks suspicious on the mammogram, you will have to have a biopsy, and this may mean waiting a few days for the results.

About one in three women who get to the biopsy stage will turn out to have cancer; this represents one in 200 of all screened women. But remember, most women with 'abnormal' mammograms will be cleared (nineteen out of twenty) and while we are throwing these figures around, it may be worth emphasising a positive aspect: 94 per cent of women *never* develop breast cancer.

[6]

What are they looking for?

THE BIOPSY AND AFTER

The purpose of a biopsy is to investigate the suspicions which have been raised by the clinical examination and the mammogram. In some cases the doctor will already know that a malignancy is present, but even if the cancer is advanced and obvious, the biopsy and subsequent analysis of tumour tissue is necessary to help formulate a view about treatment.

Generally speaking, when a woman presents herself to the doctor with symptoms she may have had for some time, it is more likely that the biopsy is going to yield bad news than when she has a biopsy as a result of an ambiguous mammogram at the screening clinic. In these latter cases, much more often than not the biopsy result will be a negative good — nothing there. Even when the biopsy does confirm the presence of a very small cancer, so early that it is defined as *in situ* rather than invasive, doctors are currently uncertain how best to deal with these lesions. The organic change is so minimal that it may never progress any further; it could even regress and ultimately disappear. This ambivalent result is plainly a major disadvantage of screening, since not only is the biopsy itself liable to cause distress but it may raise more questions than it answers. Living with uncertainty is never comfortable, but many surgeons now feel that the most ethical thing they can do in these circumstances is to adopt a 'watch and wait' policy with women to whom they cannot give a cut-and-dried answer.

Most women sent for a biopsy will be symptomatic. Already, during the clinical examination, the doctor will have made a preliminary judgement about the type of cancer she is likely to have and how far it has advanced. This is called clinical staging and is based on assessing the tumour and the state of the lymph nodes.

First the doctor feels the tumour – its size, whether it is mobile or fixed, whether it feels inflamed or solid, and how far it has affected the external appearance of the breast: for instance, by hardening the skin or dimpling it to create an effect called 'peau d'orange', reminiscent of orange peel. He will also have felt the nodes under both arms and surrounding the breasts to see whether they are enlarged and, if they are, whether they too are mobile or fixed. The condition of the nodes is an important indicator of whether the cancer has spread beyond the breast but nodes, like other lumps in the breast, can be deceptive. Sometimes they swell up and go down again for no sinister reason – or it could be that the body is successfully mobilising its immune defence system.

How the biopsy is done varies from surgeon to surgeon, and also depends on the nature of the suspect lesion. If it is an obvious lump some doctors prefer to do as wide an excision as possible in order to be sure they have extracted all the affected tissue. This really amounts to doing a lumpec-tomy at biopsy stage and could mean removing as much as one-quarter of the woman's breast, leaving her with scarring and probably a deformed outline. This is a high price to pay if the lump turns out to be benign and is really unnecessary nowadays when biopsy techniques have been so refined. Other doctors will go to great lengths to remove the smallest amount of tissue at this initial stage in an attempt to cause the least disfiguration compatible with safe surgery. Do not be afraid to ask your doctor to describe beforehand how he or she intends to do the biopsy. Those lesions which are impalpable (evident only on a mammogram and not by clinical examination) require special radiological and surgical techniques, first to locate them and then to remove a tiny amount of tissue through a minute incision. It may be necessary to follow this up with an X-ray to make certain the right piece of tissue has been removed.

The small sample of tumour tissue taken at biopsy is sent immediately to the pathologist for analysis and the results will answer most of the questions raised at the clinical examination. Pathological examination is able to define even more precisely the stage the tumour has reached and its biological character. This information helps the doctor to make a definitive diagnosis and a reasonable stab at prognosis, which is important since some types of breast cancer have a better outcome than others and this affects decisions about treatment.

Until recently it was widely accepted, and practised, that a woman going in for biopsy of a suspicious breast lump should sign a consent form beforehand, authorising the surgeon to proceed to mastectomy if analysis of the tissue confirmed a malignancy. This is now recognised as an undesirable practice, from both a medical and a humanitarian point of view. Frozen section biopsy, as this procedure is called, means that the lump is raced to the pathologist for analysis while the surgeon, his theatre team and the unconscious woman on the operating table await the verdict. Ten minutes later, the surgeon acts according to the 'yea' or 'nay' that has been delivered and a few hours later the woman wakes in her hospital bed, fearfully feeling to see whether she still has a breast.

'I somehow knew it wouldn't be there,' one young woman said to me, 'although my doctor had been swearing that it was going to be all right. I just wish he hadn't.'

This procedure is not just psychologically brutal, it is also medically unsound. The risk – once considered high – of opening a cancerous site twice is considerably outweighed by the much greater risk of making a diagnostic mistake. This race against the clock means that the pathologist cannot do extra tests which may be necessary in cases where the sample is equivocal. We will never know how many healthy breasts have been amputated on the dubious premise of better safe than sorry, but certainly doctors will admit that it has happened, too often for comfort.

I have described this procedure in some detail because although we would hope it is defunct, it is probably still being offered to women in some hospitals. If this happens to you, it is important to know that you have every right to refuse to comply. Your physical condition will not deteriorate if there is a delay of a few days at this stage, and psychologically there is much benefit to be gained from having time to absorb information and talk it over quietly in your own surroundings with those close to you.

STAGING OF BREAST CANCER

Stage 0   Carcinoma *in situ*

Stage I   Tumour is T_1 (under 2 centimetres)
Nodes are N_0 (not palpable)
and no known metastases M_0

Stage II   **Either**
Tumours are T_1
with minimal nodal involvement N_1
and no known metastases M_0
Or
Tumours are T_2 (2 to 5 cm) with or without
nodal involvement N_0 or N_1 and
no known metastases M_0

Stage III   Disease is locally spread so tumour is large, either T_3 (between 5 and 10 cm) or T_4 (more than 10 cm), probably attached to chest wall and with substantial nodal involvement N_1 or N_2 but no known metastases M_0

Stage IV   Tumour and nodes at any stage together with evidence of distant metastases M_1

As you might expect, stages I and II have the best prognosis because the disease appears to be confined to the breast and nodal involvement is very slight. The five-year survival results confirm this optimism (84 per cent for Stage I; 71 per cent for Stage II) and the usual method of treatment is surgery followed by some kind of adjuvant therapy (see chapter 9).

However, breast cancer never ceases to surprise and even when the cancer has reached Stage III – which means that the disease has spread in the breast and is usually quite obvious, suggesting that the woman has had it for some time before she reported it – it can sometimes be treated with comparative success (usually radiotherapy rather than surgery). Five-year survival figures are 48 per cent. Stage IV usually has a poor prognosis but some patients will live years longer than expected and could even die of something other than breast cancer. Sadly, it may sometimes reach that advanced stage before the woman is even aware that something is wrong.

Before we look at the treatment options available it will probably help to recapitulate some facts about breast cancer, because they have an important bearing on how the disease is managed.

First, breast cancer is not one single type of disease. Not only does it present itself in different ways, it also behaves in different ways – and often unpredictably. This is because breast cancer tumours are biologically diverse, one from another.

Second, breast cancer is not necessarily located in one single site, the breast. As the primary cancer that is where it starts, but by the time it is discovered, even when apparently very early, it may already have released cancer cells into the bloodstream to circulate and settle in distant parts of the body. These cells start up new cancer sites which may be so minute that they are quite undetectable and for a long time produce no symptoms. These are called micrometastases. It is now believed that approximately 70 per cent of breast cancers have disseminated into other parts of the body before the primary cancer is detected.

Third, although involved lymph nodes are a fairly reliable indication that cancer has already spread beyond the breast, apparently innocent nodes are not a guarantee that it has not happened anyway. About one-third of the women who did not have any lymph node involvement at the time of primary treatment do not survive beyond fifteen years, and more than one long-term study has shown that secondary breast cancer can appear even twenty years and more after the original primary.

Fourth, in the current state of the art it is still the biological nature of the tumour, rather than treatment, which determines long-term survival. This is not to say that the traditional methods of surgery and radiotherapy are no longer useful. At best they can cure the cancer (about 30 per cent of cases when it proves to be confined to the breast); at second best these methods can control the disease and make it more bearable to live with. New adjuvant treatments like chemotherapy and hormone therapy (see chapter 9) are also making it possible for women to have a better quality of life and longer disease-free periods.

The combined effect of these very telling facts produces the following conclusions: breast cancer is almost invariably a systemic disease which should, therefore, be treated systemically. Just as the disease itself is not a simple single entity, so there is no simple, single way of treating it. But conclusions don't produce answers.

Those who are most experienced in the treatment of breast cancer agree that a pooling of different skills and different disciplines offers the only hope of finding the right method of treatment for the individual woman. This is called the multidisciplinary or combined modality approach, but how the various therapies should be combined, and to what degree, and when, are still matters for research. Answers are being urgently sought in the enormous number of breast cancer trials which are currently going on all over the world.

[7]

Is your operation really necessary?

Cancer in general has been around since earliest times, as we know from traces that have been found in human remains, but it is probable that the incidence has greatly increased, perhaps particularly in the last one hundred years. There are several reasons why this should be so. More people are living longer, and cancer is primarily a disease of the old. Other factors include environmental pollution, changes in diet – in particular the modern high-fat over-processed intake – and lifestyle indulgences such as smoking and alcohol.

The history of breast cancer treatment in particular has been long, painful and controversial. We know that the Greeks and Egyptians speculated about the causes of breast cancer and we have some evidence about their methods of treatment. There are indications, for example, that breast tumours only were being cut out with knives as early as 1500 BC, and in the first century AD Celsus, a Roman writer, was advising against the more radical surgery which involves removing the chest wall muscles behind the breast tissue. This was progressive thinking then, and in some quarters today, where extended radical surgery is still being done, would be regarded as no less dangerously advanced.

The seesaw between major surgical amputation and doing little or nothing beyond cauterising the tumour has continued right down the centuries to modern times and has been well documented in Daniel de Moulin's fascinating *History of*

Breast Cancer. Anaesthetics and antiseptics were introduced little more than a hundred years ago, so it is no wonder that many women like Attossa, the wife of the Greek king, and Madame Poisson, the mother of Madame de Maintenon, preferred to endure the tumour, however terrible, rather than the barbarism of the surgeon's knife. And for those who were either brave enough to submit or perhaps too meek to protest, it was a capricious fate that awaited them.

Fanny Burney, the novelist and diarist, describes the excruciating twenty-minute operation which was performed in her sitting-room by France's leading surgeon, Dr Larrey, with six other doctors in attendance: 'When the dreadful steel was plunged into the breast — I began a scream that lasted intermittently during the whole time of the incision.' She felt the knife scraping against the breast bone and then, as the cavity was cleared, 'I bore it with all the courage I could exert and never moved, nor stopt them, nor resisted, nor remonstrated, nor spoke except once or twice, during the dressings, to say, "Messieurs, je vous plains."'[1] A tumour the size of a fist was removed but she lived healthily for another thirty years, into her late eighties. Ironically, today the medical opinion of her doctor's account is that the tumour was almost certainly benign.

THE MASTECTOMY ERA

The *classical radical* mastectomy has been the prevailing model for breast surgery ever since it was introduced in 1890 by William Halsted, an American surgeon working at the Johns Hopkins Hospital in Baltimore. It is based on the premise that breast cancer spreads centrifugally from the prime tumour in the breast through the lymph channels and nodes and only finally disseminates into other parts of the body. Therefore, runs the argument, the more tissue surrounding the breast you cut out, the better chance you have of eradicating the cancer and achieving a cure. So in addition to removing the breast tissue, the pectoral muscles supporting the breast are also cut out and there is, to use the medical phraseology, 'a radical clearance' of the axillary tissue. The effect is deforming because the patient is left concave where her breast has been removed, and hollow under the arm.

When Halsted and his colleagues realised that although they were succeeding in reducing the rates of local recurrence they were not improving survival rates, their answer was: cut some more. And so they did, often to a grossly mutilating degree because the patient lost additional tissue under the sternum, where the internal mammary nodes are located, and sometimes even part of her shoulder. No wonder such surgery has been dubbed 'heroic', but the people who deserve the medals, if they survive it, are the patients rather than the surgeons. Usually this *extended* or *super-radical* mastectomy, as it is called, was followed up by post-operative radiotherapy, which could cause severe side-effects after this traumatic surgery, particularly in the early days when dosages were far more crude than they are today.

Almost more remarkable about these two operations – and one shudders to think how many thousands of women's lives were blighted by them – is that it took almost a century and many trials before the penny finally dropped: operating on this scale was a cruel waste of time because, in the words of an early dissenter, 'If the growth had not yet been disseminated, it was unnecessary; if it had been disseminated, it was too late and useless.'[2]

Sir Geoffrey Keynes, the surgeon brother of the famous economist, Maynard, who wrote this shortly before he died in 1982, had hit upon this simple truth as long ago as 1925 when he realised that the pathology of cancer growth meant that cells could be seeded through the blood even before they were carried through the lymph glands. In the same essay he described his sense of shame and guilt when he realised that he had removed a woman's breast only to discover that the apparent carcinoma was benign. It was a lesson he could never forget and he accordingly embarked upon 'a crusade in

favour of conservative treatment, followed by careful radiotherapy to the site of origin of the growth and the axilla'. He
lectured all over the world, wrote papers and carefully
followed up his patients until the Second World War interrupted his medical career, but no one was prepared either to
listen or to learn from his experience.

Apart from a few isolated individuals who braved the scorn
of their colleagues – one was Sir Reginald Murley, a pupil of
Sir Geoffrey's at St Bartholomew's Hospital, London, who
continued his work there; another was Dr George Crile Jr in
the United States – it was not until the early eighties, and
after many trials testing various permutations of these radical
operations, that surgeons seriously began to question the
dogma that had held them in thrall since Halsted's day.
Unfortunately, some doctors are still not prepared to change
their ways or their thinking from what they learned back in
medical school days. In spite of the now conclusive evidence
that radical surgery does not improve the outcome – although
it certainly has a detrimental effect on the quality of life –
these savage mastectomies are still being performed all over
the world, not least in America, where the classical radical
remains the operation of choice. The latest notable casualty
was Nancy Reagan in 1987. (Presidential wives seem unhappily prone to breast cancer. Ten years ago, when I was writing
the first edition of this book, it was Betty Ford and Happy
Rockefeller who were making the headlines with their tear-
fully smiling comebacks.)

We do have something to be grateful for in this country.
The innate caution and conservatism of the British medical
profession has meant that doctors, while still accepting the
false premise on which the Halsted surgery was based, were
none the less concerned to reduce the mutilation, providing
they could achieve this without risking, as they saw it, the
patient's chance of cure. Two reduced forms of mastectomy
were introduced in the forties and were later submitted to
trials, with and without radiotherapy, and in comparison

with the classical radical; nevertheless, this continued to be the operation of choice for several more decades.

The *modified radical* mastectomy, sometimes called *Patey's modification* after the surgeon who devised it, is a technique which clears the axillary nodes under the arm but preserves the major pectoral muscle, thus considerably reducing the external deformity. There is no hollow below the shoulder blades and if the scar runs transversely a woman can wear a normal low-necked dress without fear of it showing. In expert hands it is a very good operation and it does almost totally eliminate the chance of local recurrence without the need for post-operative radiotherapy. However, in common with the other radical operations, it can produce the long-term side-effect of lymphoedema in the arm on the affected side (heavy arm). In this condition the arm becomes swollen with fluid which cannot drain away because the lymphatic system has been removed. It is estimated that almost half of the patients who have a radical mastectomy, even in this modified form, will suffer this complication, and in severe cases it can become painful and disabling. (See chapter 11 for exercises and suggestions for coping with it.)

The *simple* (or *total*) mastectomy, as the name suggests, involves removing the breast tissue alone, leaving both pectoral muscles intact. Depending on preference, some surgeons will also remove all the axillary nodes; others will adopt Professor Sir Patrick Forrest's technique of removing only four lower axillary nodes for sampling. Studies have now shown that providing these nodes are correctly identified and carefully analysed, their condition will give adequate guidelines for further treatment. For instance, if it appears that the lymph nodes are already affected, it may be advisable to have radiotherapy follow-up to decrease the chance of recurrence.

The obvious advantage of the simple mastectomy is that it is less traumatic and disfiguring than the radical, whether classical or modified, and there are fewer post-operative complications like lymphoedema. In the early eighties, this operation had become the treatment of choice for early breast cancer in this country. A recent survey of nearly 300 breast surgeons[3] shows that opinion has now veered strongly in favour of even more conservative surgery such as that described below. Whereas five years ago only 18 per cent of surgeons would offer a lumpectomy, today two-thirds do so.

The *partial mastectomy*, popularly known as *lumpectomy*, is also known under the names of *tylectomy, local, wide* or *wedge excision*. This involves removing the lump alone with not much more than one centimetre of surrounding tissue, the aim being to cause as little mutilation as possible compatible with removing all the visible malignancy. It is usually, but not always, supported by radiotherapy to inhibit local recurrence, and lymph node sampling, using the Forrest technique, can be done at the same time. Ten years ago lumpectomy was regarded as an experimental – if not downright dangerous – procedure, and most surgeons refused to do it for reasons already explained in this chapter; they feared they would leave some cancer behind or that there might be other undetected sites in the breast.

Today, trials have conclusively demonstrated that as far as long-term survival is concerned, there is no difference between a total and a partial mastectomy.[4] In effect, what surgery does is to deal with the immediate problem of eradicating the primary tumour and preventing its spread in the breast. This is important because tumours that are neglected will almost certainly ulcerate and may progress to such a point that they become inoperable. At the very worst they will fungate, a condition as unpleasant and malodorous as the word suggests, and the condition becomes extremely painful and irreversible. The point to remember is that a small tumour can be controlled by a small operation, hence the importance of early detection.

The modern thinking behind surgery for early breast cancer has three main objectives: the first is to achieve local control, by removing tumour tissue in the breast and surrounding area, should it exist; the second is to dissect out the axillary nodes for analysis because it is their status which will determine whether and what further treatment is necessary; and the third is to make sure that all available tumour tissue is submitted to proper histological analysis. Until recently, the arguments against lumpectomy were that none of these objectives could be achieved with any degree of certainty. However, since mammography has become a routine part of the diagnostic procedure it is much less likely that other cancers will be missed; use of the Forrest technique to sample axillary nodes disposes of the second objection; and surgeons can be sure there will be enough tumour for complete analysis providing they remove the lump with an adequate margin of surrounding tissue.

What surgery cannot do is to control disease which has already become systemic – in other words has escaped from the breast into other parts of the body. If it has reached this stage – and this is true for 70 per cent of diagnosed breast cancer – a woman will need some kind of further treatment (see chapter 9). For the foreseeable future – and certainly while breast cancer remains unpreventable and not invariably curable by other means – there will always be some women who, for medical reasons, will need to have a total mastectomy. Briefly, they are these: when the tumour is large (over 4 centimetres), or located behind the nipple, or there are several cancer sites in the breast.

There are other non-medical reasons which may make a woman prefer the option of mastectomy to lumpectomy. For example, her breasts may be small in relation to the size of the lump, so that a lumpectomy could actually be more disfiguring than a mastectomy. Other women may feel psychologically insecure about a lumpectomy. They fear that the cancer may not all have come out, whatever the doctor may say to reassure them. These and other considerations which may influence a woman's choices and decisions about treatment are discussed in greater depth in chapter 17.

The mastectomy era is not yet quite at an end, although there is now a distinct and realistic hope that by the end of the century this particular amputation, with all its attendant suffering, will have become a rarity, reserved only for unusual cases. Modified breast surgery to control the local disease will probably continue to be the treatment of choice for most women, even though it is now possible to achieve the same results with radiotherapy (see chapter 8) and perhaps other treatments with similar potential are already being developed. Saving the breast does not necessarily enable a woman to live longer, but it can certainly improve the quality of her life.

[8]

Conservation or reconstruction

CONSERVATION – LUMPECTOMY

Most women want to keep their breast, if this is at all possible. Not so many realise that there are treatment choices open to them. Now that lumpectomy has been shown to be equally effective as mastectomy in the treatment of early breast cancer, every woman diagnosed at this stage should be aware that this is an option she can consider – provided, of course, that there are no sound medical reasons in her case which might militate against it. *Conservative* surgery, as it is called, is a lumpectomy usually followed up by radiotherapy. The aim is to minimise deforming and scarring the breast, so the operation obviously produces better results when the lump is small. Usually the upper limit is a diameter of three centimetres, but it can be larger in women with bigger breasts and still achieve an aesthetic outcome.

Until recently the majority of surgeons gave no choice to their patients, and mastectomy was the only 'safe' treatment on offer. You had to be a very brave and determined woman to insist on being told about other treatments, let alone request that you be given one of them. Lumpectomies have in fact been performed for many years, either by doctors who were already intellectually convinced that they were effective or as part of a clinical trial where patients are randomly allocated to different treatments which are then carefully compared for outcome, side-effects and long-term results.

Some of the patients entered without their knowledge into

a trial would have been pleasurably surprised to be told by their surgeon that they needed only the small operation. They might not have been so pleased had they realised that the decision rested not with their doctor but on a randomised computer instruction. Many thousands of women have been entered into such trials without their knowledge and consent, but it is thanks to their unwitting participation all over the world that doctors now know for sure that there is no significant difference in long-term outcome between mastectomy and lumpectomy. (See chapter 17 for a discussion of the ethical implications of randomised clinical trials.)

A recent survey of nearly 300 surgeons[1] has revealed that these findings have made the majority change their practice quite considerably. Whereas in 1983 only 18 per cent of surgeons were prepared to do a lumpectomy, today more than two-thirds offer it and say, moreover, that they are willing to discuss the pros and cons of the various treatments. Clearly this is an advance but the time they are able to give each patient is still very short, around ten minutes on average, and very few follow this up with written information. This matters, because the topic is complicated and technical and people need time to absorb its import and discuss it with those who are close to them before they can truly be ready to make an informed decision.

CONSERVATION – RADIOTHERAPY

Radiotherapy is the treatment of disease by radiation energy. It is designed to destroy tumour cells while leaving healthy tissue relatively unaffected, but whatever slight damage may occur to normal cells will be repaired fairly quickly. These days, the type of energy used is most often a high-energy (megavoltage) X-ray beam, which in skilful hands, where the amount and frequency of the dose are carefully monitored, causes minimum reaction. This energy is similar to, but much more powerful than, the low-energy beams produced by X-rays done for diagnostic purposes.

There are almost as many variations in technique as there are radiotherapists to administer the treatment and women who need it. Each woman is different in shape, size and state of health at the time of treatment. Tumours, as we have seen, also vary greatly in type, size and location. Those which are slow-growing are less sensitive to radiation and may therefore require more prolonged or higher dosage. Others which grow more rapidly tend also to respond better to radiotherapy, which may be administered as the sole primary treatment without surgery.

Radiotherapy can be used to supplement surgery, both on the tumour site and in the axilla to eradicate any lingering vestiges of malignancy in the lymph nodes. It can also be used as a treatment on its own; this has been particularly popular in France, possibly because French women have been more vocal about and resistant to losing their breasts. In this country irradiation as a primary treatment without surgery has tended to be reserved for advanced cancer where the tumour mass is large and spreading and deemed inoperable.

However, sixty years after Sir Geoffrey Keynes's pioneering work with radium needles, a very similar operation is now being done at Guy's Hospital in London for early breast cancer. The lump is removed and radioactive wires are then passed into the breast and kept there for three to four days to irradiate the area of malignancy. Conventional radiotherapy will be given to the surrounding tissue, particularly in the axilla to lessen the chance of local recurrence. Variations on this treatment are currently being tested in several centres in North America and compared with conventional surgery. Already the opinion is being cautiously expressed that 'primary radiation therapy appears to be a reasonable alternative to mastectomy for women with early breast cancer.'[2]

Given the acknowledged success of this treatment, why is it not more readily available in this country? One reason is that inserting the wires (interstitial implant, as it is called) requires not only a high degree of skill and care from the radiotherapist but also close co-operation with the surgeon and other members of the medical team. Time, commitment and expertise are all essential – and are not always present in sufficient amounts in the one overloaded hospital department. It is also important that the woman understands the implications of the treatment. If it works, she will have preserved her breast and it will continue to look pretty good. Sometimes, though, the skin texture, colour and general appearance of the breast may gradually alter and she should be aware of this possibility. She should also be warned that were the cancer to recur in the breast (and this can happen in a small minority of cases even after radiotherapy) she would then have to have a mastectomy. This is not comfortable knowledge to possess but if, as patients, we want to take part in the decision-making process about treatment, we must be ready to take responsibility for our decisions.

RADIOTHERAPY – TREATMENT AND SIDE-EFFECTS

The radiotherapist (doctor) draws up an individual treatment plan for each patient, and this needs careful preparation. Several visits may be necessary to what is called a 'simulator', where X-ray pictures are taken to decide on the area for treatment. The skin is then marked with indelible ink to pinpoint the site, and before each dose of treatment, felt pens will circumscribe the margins. These marks must not be washed off during the weeks of treatment. The treatment itself from the machine is very brief, but what does take time is the positioning beforehand to ensure that the beam is accurately directed. The radiographer (technician) leaves the room while the machine is on, but she watches you constantly throughout the treatment and she can hear you and respond if you want to speak to her.

The course of treatment may last anything from four to six or more weeks, five days a week, and it is quite normal to feel tired and possibly nauseous and a bit low during this time. Side-effects vary with individuals. Everyone suffers some degree of redness, which looks like mild sunburn, but people with fair skin may feel more soreness. Before the treatment starts the radiographer will explain how you should look after your skin during this period, but here are some general rules.

The area being treated should not be washed at all, nor should you apply any kind of creams or perfumes, because these too could cause soreness. A good baby powder is safe, providing there is no 'weepiness' on the skin, and sprinkling this liberally should help relieve any itching or discomfort, but if there are any problems, stop using it and ask the radiographer for advice. It is also a good idea to wear loose clothing and probably no bra so that there is no pressure on the area being treated. Do not expose the treated area to the sun, either during the treatment or for a few weeks afterwards, as it will remain sensitive for a while. You will not lose your head hair as a result of radiotherapy to the breast, but it will fall out from your armpit and it is important neither to apply deodorant nor attempt to shave there. If you have any problems at all, do not endure them in stoical silence but report them immediately to the radiographer or the doctor so that the appropriate action can be taken.

Sometimes doctors are not sufficiently aware of the time and effort it takes their patients to keep this daily appointment during treatment. Because you look all right and are probably getting yourself to and from the hospital, your family and friends may also assume that you are coping pretty well. In fact you will undoubtedly need some support and cosseting during this time. Make sure you eat well, try and get as much rest as possible, and do not overdo things, either at work or in the home.

BREAST RECONSTRUCTION

Basically this means replacing the amputated breast by some form of implant, natural or artificial, which is placed on the chest wall under the breast skin either at the time of the mastectomy or a few months or even years later. On the whole it is easier to do at the primary stage but some doctors prefer to wait, not just because they think they can achieve a better cosmetic result but also because they consider it is important for women to be given the chance to think through what reconstruction means.

This represents a significant change in medical attitudes, one that has come about because of the increased recognition that a mutilating operation like a mastectomy can have a detrimental effect on a patient's psychological condition. Until recently most doctors were very negative about offering breast reconstruction. Either they thought it inadvisable because of the possibility of local recurrence – a fear which has now been proved groundless, because if it should happen the implant can easily be removed – or, more judgementally, they dismissed it as a foolish vanity not to be indulged.

When I was researching for this book in the mid seventies there were hardly any doctors offering the operation to patients who had breast cancer, although they were prepared to do it, if asked, on patients with benign breast disease. Only one doctor was prepared to discuss his work with me and introduce me to his patients, but his colleagues regarded him with suspicion and tried to dismiss his excellent results on the grounds that they were too selective. Even now, only about 5 per cent of women undergoing a mastectomy follow it up with a breast reconstruction, a suspiciously low percentage compared with the proportion of women who are known to experience distress at losing their breast. The survey of 300 surgeons referred to on p. 78 revealed that the majority of those doing mastectomies did not offer reconstruction to their patients, but that is hardly a surprising finding, since these are the very same doctors who are adhering to an operation which is rapidly going out of favour. Their conservatism is proven and means that they will be less rather than more likely to consider reconstruction as an option. It is important, however, for women to know that this option exists and that it is neither freakish nor frivolous to want to consider it.

Many women feel intuitively that they need time to mourn the loss of their breast and come to terms with the situation before deciding whether they want to replace it. This is a reaction which should be respected, and since doctors who work in this particular field have been sensitised to the needs of their patients, the offer will not be pressed. There will be other women, however, who will want a replacement at once. They need careful counselling to make sure they understand that it is unlikely to be an exact replica of their lost breast. Given this precondition – and provided, of course, that it is medically feasible – their request should be met.

It can't be stressed too strongly that it is most important that women asking for breast reconstruction should clearly understand what it can and cannot do for them. There is no point in entertaining false hopes, either physically or psychologically. If, for instance, a marriage is in a troubled, unstable state, restoring a breast is not necessarily going to restore the relationship. On the other hand, if a woman's sense of self-esteem and femininity is very much tied up with her body image, it will obviously enhance her confidence if she feels that her shape has not been changed too much. The reconstruction may not achieve much more than a breast mound, but this may be sufficient to make her feel at least at ease with her external, clothed appearance.

There is a certain Amazonian view expressed by some feminists which condemns this attitude, taking the line that it is weak and inauthentic of a woman to believe she can be whole only if she is twin-breasted. To imagine this, runs the argument, is to swallow the male view of sexuality and live supinely in a male reflection.[3] Women, urge the hardline feminists, should be unashamed of their breastlessness – indeed, positively assert it, and by so doing reject the men who reject them. Obviously this means rejecting any substitutes like breast reconstruction or a breast prosthesis (artificial breast). While for some women this may be possible and indeed prove a cathartic way of overcoming their grief, for others it will sound as harsh and judgemental in its own way as the traditional, peculiarly Anglo-Saxon and invariably male doctor who regards the female breast as no more than an appendage which outgrows its use and loses its appeal as its owner ages. According to this view, whereas some sympathy may be felt for a young woman's distress, the middle-aged and old are supposed to be beyond concern about their sexual relationships or even their appearance.

Both these points of view are extreme and, in the final analysis, profoundly unimaginative and uncaring. It is certainly true that a woman is more than the sum of her sexual characteristics and does not live and have her being only through her sexual role, yet many women who do not think about themselves in a strongly sexual context none the less feel a deep sense of violation at the prospect of losing a breast. It has been an intimate part of them all their adult life, and now it is being wrested from them.

There is also an important practical consideration to take into account, one which is all too easily overlooked. The after-effects of a mastectomy can be physically most uncomfortable, particularly if the woman has large, heavy breasts. Her balance will be affected and she may have difficulty finding a prosthesis which fits her. And even those many women who do adjust quite successfully to wearing a prosthesis may still be nervous about losing it in embarrassing circumstances – swimming or dancing, for instance. You have to be very self-confident indeed, or flat-chested, to go about your everyday life with one side of your chest deflated. You are certainly no less of a real woman on the inside if you decide you would prefer to continue looking like a complete woman on the outside.

Studies both here and in America have shown that women who are offered breast reconstruction at the time of their mastectomy and given the opportunity to choose from the following options – have it at the same time, wait a while, or turn it down – are all ultimately better psychologically adjusted to their illness, whichever option they pick, than women given no choice. One particularly important study notes that 'the most striking feature' of offering this choice to women was their 'general satisfaction' and gratitude, irrespective of their final decision.[4] 'It would certainly seem', note the authors, 'that having a degree of control helped the women to adapt well.'

METHODS OF BREAST RECONSTRUCTION

There are currently five standard ways of reconstructing a breast; which one is chosen depends to a large extent on the position of the tumour, what kind of mastectomy has been done, and the state of the surrounding tissue. Some surgeons would prefer to wait for a few months before doing the reconstruction to allow the remaining tissue to recover, particularly if the mastectomy was followed up by radiotherapy. The surgeon will discuss with the patient the details of the operation, the complications she may have and the kind of cosmetic results she can realistically expect. Plainly, the aim is to simulate the lost breast and match it as closely as possible with the one that remains, but a perfect result is not always possible, even in the most skilled hands. Sometimes it may be necessary to reduce the size of the healthy breast to achieve balance, and it may not always be possible to reproduce the nipple, so the end result may be more of a 'breast mound' than a breast.

Simple augmentation: a silicone prosthesis, usually a soft, malleable gel contained in a thin transparent silicone envelope, is inserted in a deep pocket between the pectoral muscle and the chest wall.

Tissue expansion: a purpose-built tissue expander is inserted into a deep pocket (as above) at the time of the mastectomy. It is gradually distended until it matches the other breast; then it is replaced by a silicone prosthesis. The process usually takes about eight weeks and can be quite painful and disabling while it lasts, but it does have a good cosmetic result.

Local flaps: some abdominal skin is taken up into the

mastectomy area and combined with an internal silicone prosthesis.

Latissimis dorsi myocutaneous flap: muscle is taken from the back and augmented if necessary, with an internal silicone prosthesis.

Rectus abdominus myocutaneous flap: fat is taken from the omentum, an apron of tissue that hangs in front of the bowel to protect it from injury, and rolled up into the mastectomy area without being severed from its blood supply. This is a major operation but it apparently has excellent cosmetic results.

There is always some risk that a silicone prosthesis will form a hard shell due to leakage of the gel. There are various ways of counteracting this disadvantage, the best now being to insert the prosthesis under the muscle rather than directly under the skin, as used to be done. If a woman wants a nipple as well, this can be made using skin from the vulva or the top of the leg. This is usually done by a plastic surgeon whereas the breast reconstructions can be done by general surgeons, preferably those who specialise in breast surgery.

Breast reconstruction is not going to make you quite as good as new but it does make many women feel more confident and secure, not only in the way they look to the world but in their own outlook on life. Carol Brickman, who bravely wrote a full-page article for *The Times* about her operation and why she decided to have it,[5] told me that she was glad she had to wait eighteen months before the surgeon would do the operation: 'It helped me to adjust and it gave me a chance to look at myself and become aware that I was a risk case. If you rectify something too quickly you don't have time to think it through.' Other research[6] suggests that for some women at least, immediate reconstruction is better – particularly for those who are worried about their partner's reaction.

What this indicates is that women vary enormously in their needs and responses. They certainly should not be made to feel guilty for caring about their appearance or worrying about their sexual relationships. These concerns affect the quality of their life, so it is important that they be given the opportunity to air them and talk them through with an experienced counsellor before deciding on their treatment option.

[9]

What else can they do?

As we now know, breast cancer is a complex disease involving a multitude of factors such as a woman's age, her menstrual history and status, the kind of tumour, the stage it is at and the initial treatment which is prescribed, all interacting and affecting the ultimate outcome. In addition to the clinical variability of the disease, there are all sorts of half-guessed-at but basically unquantifiable environmental and lifestyle influences also playing their part which make it quite impossible to predict with certainty who will benefit from what treatment regimen. Despite the numerous clinical trials which have been going on worldwide for over thirty years, doctors remain fundamentally baffled by the vagaries of this disease, and its unpredictability greatly complicates their task of explaining treatment options to the patient.

Take the fact, for instance, that 30 per cent of the women who are diagnosed node-negative at the time of primary treatment – and are, therefore, deemed to have a good prognosis – will none the less suffer recurrence of the disease within five years. *How* this happens is known: it is because breast cancer sometimes bypasses the lymph nodes, which are the body's sentinels, and slips into the system via the blood-stream. But *why* it should happen, or how it can be prevented, is still not known. What the researchers are currently seeking are more reliable biochemical markers to indicate those women who are most at risk of recurrence. For instance, changes in the blood, urine or other evidence of metabolic transformation are all possible bio-markers but how to identify their specific relevance for breast cancer is both the key and a mystery at the present time.

One bio-marker which has been identified and is very useful for guiding doctors in their decisions about additional treatments is what is called the *oestrogen receptor* status of the tumour. At least 70 per cent of breast tumours contain molecules called oestrogen receptor protein. If the tumour contains this protein it is described as oestrogen-positive and the more it has, the higher the probability that the patient will respond well to either hormone therapy or cytotoxic drugs (chemotherapy). Correspondingly, it seems that oestrogen-negative tumours are not so sensitive and treatment, therefore, is not so effective.

There are two situations where doctors will consider prescribing treatments in addition to surgery and radiotherapy. The first is when there seems to be no obvious spread beyond the breast and lymph nodes, yet the pathology and stage of the tumour suggest that the cancer is highly likely to recur. The purpose of extra treatment at this stage will be to destroy small, undetected cancer sites in other parts of the body (micrometastases). The second situation inviting additional treatment is when the cancer has definitely come back and there is a need to control the spread.

There have been many clinical trials of these various adjuvant therapies, as they are more correctly termed (definition on page 91) and, broadly speaking, this is the consensus view which has emerged. Where there is a primary cancer, chemotherapy cures a small proportion of pre-menopausal women who have node-positive cancer; post-menopausal women, also with node-positive primary cancer, are better served by hormone therapy. This usually takes the form of tamoxifen (brand name Novaldex), an anti-oestrogen drug. Doctors are very divided about using tamoxifen in pre-menopausal women or prescribing any form of adjuvant therapy for node-negative women, but almost everyone agrees that chemotherapy is useless for post-menopausal women.

However, the situation changes when it is a matter of treating secondary cancer. Here the choice of treatment will depend more on the cancer site than on the woman's age. Hormone treatments work better for women who have positive receptors or slow-growing tumours which are located in the bone or soft tissue. Chemotherapy appears to be more effective for women with receptor-negative tumours or metastases in the lungs or liver.

Doctors, quite properly, do not want to give treatments to women who feel well and show no signs of systemic disease unless they can be sure they are going to be beneficial in the long term – that is to say, will definitely prolong life or, at the very least, significantly delay the return of disease. They also need to know which treatment is likely to have the best results for patients who clearly already have systemic disease. So how can doctors assess the various treatments which, though available, may still be at the comparison stage? Should they indeed be entering their own patients into the trials comparing these treatments, in order, as the researchers maintain, to hasten the progress towards a more certain state of knowledge?

To give an example of the kind of dilemma that faces the ordinary clinician looking after his various breast cancer patients and wondering what to give them: the results of four trials testing tamoxifen and various combinations of chemotherapy on node-negative patients were recently published in the *New England Journal of Medicine*, together with two completely conflicting commentaries on how the results should be interpreted.[1] To boil down the argument to its basic essentials, one author disagrees with the way the risks and benefits have been measured and believes that there is no justification for entering so many apparently cancer-free women into these treatment regimens.[2] He points out, for good measure, that the severity of the side-effects in a couple of the chemotherapy trials has been glossed over: some women were wretchedly ill and a few even died from the treatment. The other author believes the side-effects to be negligible and the results so significant and in favour of these therapies 'that all women with newly diagnosed localized invasive breast cancer can and should be offered some form of systemic treatment within or outside of a clinical trial'.[3]

If two scientists can reach such opposing interpretations from the same sets of results, how can the ordinary doctor − let alone the unfortunate woman who is more than likely to be devoid of medical knowledge − be expected to make rational decisions about treatments? But decisions do have to be made, and they have to be based on more than medical evidence. Quality of life and a woman's personal expectations and needs must also come into the equation. (More about this in part three).

A FEW DEFINITIONS

This is perhaps the moment to define the differences between the terms 'adjuvant systemic therapy', 'symptomatic therapy' and 'combined modality therapy', all of which are used frequently in the medical literature but should also be understood by women if they want to have a better appreciation of the various treatment options.

Adjuvant means additional or auxiliary and refers to any treatment, such as hormone therapy or chemotherapy, which is used at the same time as the primary cancer is first treated in a curative way − that is to say by surgery, possibly combined with radiotherapy.

Systemic means that the therapy is treating the whole bodily system, not just the site of the primary cancer, on the assumption that the cancer has already spread.

Symptomatic defines therapy which is applied when there are symptoms of recurrent cancer. Breast cancer can spread to the bones and various organs in the body and the treatment which is chosen will be whatever is most appropriate, the aim being first to control the cancer and, when that ceases to be possible, to palliate the pain and discomfort caused by secondary tumours.

Combined modality means that the different therapies – surgery, radiotherapy, hormone therapy and chemotherapy – are used either sequentially or in various permutations to treat the disease at both primary and secondary stages.

MORE ABOUT HORMONE (ENDOCRINE) THERAPY

Ever since a certain Mr Beatson, a Scottish surgeon, discovered in 1885 that by removing the ovaries of two of his patients who had advanced breast cancer he was able to halt the disease for a considerable period, doctors have realised that there is a close relationship between breast cancer and sex hormones. What it is exactly and how best it can be exploited to improve the patient's condition is still, today, not clearly understood. The basic theory is that many, if not all, breast cancers are hormone-dependent.

In the old days hormone therapy consisted exclusively of removing various hormone-producing organs, starting with the ovaries (oophorectomy), then, if the cancer recurred, removing the adrenal glands (adrenalectomy), and finally the pituitary gland (hypophysectomy), a major and traumatic operation. Nowadays these two latter operations are no longer performed because there are medical alternatives which are equally effective and achieve the same results without the drastic surgery. The oophorectomy continues to be a very common procedure for pre-menopausal women but it is now usually done with radiotherapy rather than surgery. This is because there are several studies to show that some patients who fail to respond to tamoxifen will do well with an oophorectomy. Tamoxifen is a complex drug which has a quite different action on the body's metabolism as compared with the simple removal of ovarian function, achieved by an oophorectomy. In some women tamoxifen actually increases the oestrogen level, even though it is called an anti-oestrogen.

An oophorectomy, whether surgical or radiation-induced, is a relatively simple procedure, which probably explains why surgeons have tended to be very casual about its major side-effect – an early menopause. 'By the way, expect the change of life,' is the way one woman told me her surgeon chose to communicate this important piece of information to her, volunteering it as a throwaway line over his shoulder as he left the room. To a woman, already devastated by the knowledge of her cancer, this can be a severe extra cause of distress. She has to accept that this is the end of her fertile life and she may have been wanting to have children or complete her family. Even if this is not in her mind, the burden of coping with hot flushes, increased anxiety and other meno-pausal symptoms at a low ebb in her life deserves at the least sympathy and understanding.

Here is one of the many occasions where the nurse counsel-lor can be tremendously helpful. Apart from her professional training, she is another woman who can identify with these particular problems at the same human level. Unfortunately, there are not yet enough of these specially trained nurses and some surgeons are still unconvinced that they need their services. (More about the role of these nurses in chapter 11).

Although doctors are not in agreement about the benefits of tamoxifen for pre-menopausal women, there is now no doubt that it is very effective for many post-menopausal women, even for some whose tumour is oestrogen-negative. A recently published overview of the many trials[4] shows that tamoxifen given as an adjuvant therapy to post-menopausal women who have some involved axillary nodes significantly improves their chance of living longer without recurrence of the disease. Whether it improves their long-term survival – that is, beyond ten years – is still open to doubt, but these results are good enough to justify prescribing tamoxifen to all older women who meet these criteria.

It is easy to be dazzled – by figures and so-called significant results which, in truth, usually represent very small percent-age improvements – into believing that taking a certain drug will guarantee cure. Doctors get dazzled too, excited by the enthusiasm of their colleagues, and may 'oversell' a particular therapy to their patients without making it clear that success cannot be guaranteed in every case, just that there is a better chance of achieving it. To the individual woman that chance may be well worth grasping at, particularly if the risks and side-effects are not too great.

A major advantage of tamoxifen as compared to chemo-therapy is that it is non-toxic and produces relatively fewer and less severe side-effects. Hot flushes if you are pre-menopausal, a tendency to put on weight and vaginal dis-charge are probably the most that women will suffer. Very rarely a more severe side-effect has been reported, like thrombo-embolism. It is also easy to take – tablets every day for at least two years after the primary treatment. All in all, tamoxifen marks an important advance in the treatment of breast cancer and ranks as one of the major achievements of the last decade, justifying the many trials that have been run to test it. But, to echo a respected American doctor,[5] there is no further reason to be running trials of tamoxifen with a placebo. It has taken its place in the breast cancer pharmaco-poeia and future trials should be based on comparing it with other treatments for specific conditions.

Tamoxifen is a versatile drug. Apart from its value as an adjuvant therapy for primary breast cancer and as a first line of attack for women with secondary cancer, there is also a view that it may work as a prophylactic treatment for women who are at high risk of contracting breast cancer. The Imperial Cancer Research Fund is currently running a trial enlisting 4,000 women over the age of fifty known to have at least three high-risk factors, half of whom will be taking tamoxifen every day for five years. If the trial achieves its aim of securing a 50 per cent reduction in breast cancer, it will certainly have proved its value for this vulnerable group of women. Volunteers have been recruited from screening and breast clinics and the trial co-ordinators emphasise that their co-operation has been obtained on the basis of fully informed, written consent.

MORE ABOUT CHEMOTHERAPY

Over the past twenty years, cytotoxic (anti-cancer) drugs have been used to an ever-increasing extent. Initially, single drugs were used; then, as understanding grew of the way they worked on the tumour and on the body generally, various combinations were and are being tested with the dual aim of improving response and reducing the side-effects, some of which can be deeply unpleasant. Length of regime is also being tested and this is very important in relation to side-effects because the longer the drugs are administered, the more toxic the patient becomes.

At first chemotherapy was used to treat advanced cancer with the aim of securing good remission for patients because at this stage the most it can do is control the disease, not cure it. Now, however, chemotherapy is increasingly prescribed for many women as an adjuvant systemic therapy for primary breast cancer, starting immediately after their surgery or radiotherapy. Here the aim is to improve the chance of survival and it seems, judging from the recently published results cited earlier in this chapter,[6] that it succeeds to some extent. A review of thirty-one trials[7] has shown that chemotherapy works better for the younger pre-menopausal women and that among their ranks there will be a significantly higher number of survivors after five years. Whether they will go on to live longer altogether than untreated women has not yet been proven.

Chemotherapy as an adjuvant systemic treatment works by attacking the cells which have escaped into the bloodstream from the primary cancer. Although there is still a great deal of uncertainty about the exact relationship of these seeded cells to the primary tumour, some researchers think that when this tumour is removed from the breast any such micrometastases (minute spreads) which might otherwise have lain dormant are stimulated into growth. Therefore, goes the argument for chemotherapy, if you can administer the right dose at this early stage, when these residual cancer cells are fast-growing and very responsive to drugs, you may be able to knock them all off before they have a chance to develop.

Unfortunately, chemotherapy has a way of attacking some normal cells as well, in particular those which divide more frequently than others. The blood, hair follicles, bone marrow and mouth are all sites for these particular rapid-growth normal cells, and this explains why side-effects mostly affect these parts of the body. Hair loss, extreme nausea, vomiting, diarrhoea, cystitis and numbness in the fingertips are all characteristic effects. Loss of white cells in the blood means that you may feel very tired and are more susceptible to infection, so blood counts have to be taken regularly and if necessary you may have to have a blood transfusion or take antibiotics. It is not surprising, therefore, that many women also suffer emotional and psychological side-effects such as depression and loss of libido (sex drive).

For these reasons British doctors, to their credit, have been much more cautious than their American counterparts about prescribing chemotherapy, particularly the more aggressive and long-lasting regimes. It is worth knowing, too, that not everyone suffers all these side-effects at the same time or to the same degree, and they do cease once the chemotherapy ends. Many British doctors are now actually reverting to single-agent chemotherapy because they find that the new drugs – Mitozantrone, for instance – are just as effective while producing far less severe side-effects. You should not feel any diffidence about asking your doctor to discuss these different options in chemotherapy with you.

SYMPTOMATIC RADIOTHERAPY

Local recurrence is what happens when small, imperceptible deposits of cancer cells, left unwittingly in the skin or other tissue near the primary tumour at the time of the first operation, become activated. It usually manifests as small external growths along the scar line or as internal lumps. Local recurrence is a development of the primary cancer and is, therefore, a form of secondary (metastatic) disease.

Unfortunately, between 5 and 10 per cent of women will suffer local recurrence whatever first treatment they receive, but providing it is reported immediately it can usually be effectively removed with a short course of radiotherapy. All the same, it still comes as an unpleasant shock to the unfortunate women who suffer it, especially if they had been misleadingly reassured by their surgeon after the original operation, as so many are, that the cancer has been entirely removed. Of course, that is what everyone hopes for, and for many it will be true, but not for everyone . Women should be aware of this possibility and not be lulled into a false sense of security. Phrases like 'We've caught it in time', or 'It was just on the turn', or 'We've managed to get it all out' should be banned from the doctors' vocabulary.

Medical opinion differs considerably about the best way of preventing local recurrence. The traditional methods have been variations of surgery combined with adjuvant radiotherapy: for instance, either a simple mastectomy or a lumpectomy supported by radiotherapy, or a radical mastectomy accompanied either by radical radiotherapy or, with the same effect, complete surgical clearance of the axillary nodes. None of these methods is totally satisfactory because they cause the lymph nodes to be removed before establishing whether they are involved. It is not certain what effect their removal has on a woman's immune system but it certainly heightens her risk of developing lymphoedema in the arm on the side of the treated breast – a distressing and irreversible side-effect.

Since no treatment can guarantee 100 per cent safety from local recurrence, some doctors prefer to adopt a 'watch and wait' policy using radiotherapy only if and when local recurrence does happen. An alternative is to use the Forrest technique of node sampling when doing either a simple mastectomy or a lumpectomy, and then follow it up with selective radiotherapy for those women who appear to run a greater risk of local recurrence.

Distant disease occurs when the cancer appears as secondaries in other parts of the body. Radiotherapy can be used very effectively to relieve pain, particularly when there is cancer in the bones, and to shrink tumours.

Whatever the treatment chosen, it is now an accepted principle that great care should be taken not to destroy the body's defence mechanisms needlessly; hence one reason for conservative surgery is not to do too much damage to local tissue. Similarly with radiotherapy: it should be adopted with discrimination and only because it is felt to be the best way of dealing with the particular tumour, or it is necessary to treat a local recurrence. Fewer doctors now use it as an automatic post-operative routine because they worry about the long-term consequences of destroying adequately functioning lymph nodes. Although there is still much to discover about how the lymph nodes and other defence mechanisms in the body do their work, it is clear that regional lymph nodes (those in close proximity to a tumour) will respond immunologically – that is to say, fight the tumour, at least for a while, presumably until they are overcome by its growing strength and size.

With a systemic treatment like chemotherapy, even greater care is required because the harm that could be caused by injudiciously reducing the body's defences is more widespread and more insidious. There is now plenty of evidence to show that long regimes have no advantage over shorter ones.

Immunology has a long way to go, and much remains to be discovered before it can be regarded as a useful therapeutic arm of medicine, but even in its present embryonic stage it sounds a suitably cautious note for those who, in their enthusiasm for man-made remedies, forget that nature too has a vital role to play in the curing and healing process.

[10]

Mind and body

FEELINGS – AT THE BEGINNING

A diagnosis of breast cancer is a shattering event for any woman. The fear of malignancy will have been simmering within her ever since she, or the mammogram, discovered the lump, and she will have experienced mounting tension and distress as she went through the various diagnostic procedures. This fear will have been intensified if hospital staff appear indifferent to her feelings or too busy to talk to her. Now she has to face the reality: cancer is in her body and it threatens her life.

None of us can predict how we will react to a life-threatening crisis until it happens, nor can we easily imagine how we will carry on afterwards. It seems common for people to be overwhelmed by a flood of conflicting feelings, often starting with incredulity, a sense of 'This can't be happening to me. I'm not this person being told this news.' Many women say that just hearing the word 'cancer' blotted out anything further the doctor may have told them. Quite literally, they did not hear. Fear of death blankets them and soon other fears creep in under this all-pervading emotion; the fear of mutilation, of pain, of rejection, of humiliation, the numbing dread of not knowing what to expect.

'I felt dazed and unbelieving. This couldn't be happening to me. The world felt spongy, sort of damped down and unreal. Everyone seemed a long way away, their voices muffled. I'll never know to this day how I drove myself home,' is how one woman described her initial reaction. Like so many others she had gone to the breast clinic on her own, completely unprepared for the bad news awaiting her.

It is appalling how often doctors, even today when more of them profess themselves aware of the psychological stress a verdict of cancer induces, still seem unable to communicate the bad news in a manner that is other than brusque and curt, in some cases almost suggesting that the condition is the patient's fault.

A bleak announcement that 'the breast will have to come off' is cruel beyond belief, yet it has frequently been reported to me as the way a woman was told about her cancer. To some degree this is explained by the average surgeon's mechanistic view of disease: he defines the problem, measures the malignancy and cuts it out with the knife. He has removed the tumour: *ipso facto* 'cure' has been achieved, and with that act he believes he has fulfilled his responsibility towards his patient.

Perhaps, too, he has a problem with his own emotions. In medical school he was taught to cultivate detachment and not allow his feelings to surface for fear they might cloud his clinical judgement. He believes he cannot afford to let himself become too involved with the anxieties and concerns of his patients, otherwise how would he get through the day? He knows his patients have problems – indeed, he would have to be grossly insensitive if he did not – but he is uncertain how to acknowledge them or handle them positively, especially if he happens himself to have very negative feelings about cancer, and many doctors and nurses do.

Health professionals need help too, to come to terms with their feelings by talking them through and admitting their own fears and vulnerability, in particular their sense of helplessness and frustration. Ideally they would do this with a trained counsellor, but this kind of support is not easily available within or outside the NHS. Now that there is increasing pressure to speed up patient through-put and reduce costs, it is even less likely to be offered in the future.

Since this book is written mainly for women, it concentrates on the feelings and difficulties they experience in communicating with their doctors and others who are caring for them. Many of these problems are, sadly, doctor-induced and, therefore, even harder to handle from the woman's point of view. There are, however, some good books written with insight and concern by doctors for doctors with the aim of helping them to understand themselves better and thus to function more effectively as compassionate human beings. A few of the best are listed in the Resources section because although they are useful for patients to help them understand why doctors so often behave as they do, they might have an even more positive effect if they were read by the doctors themselves.

Another familiar type of defensive behaviour is for the doctor to retreat behind euphemisms or bland assurances that all will be well. Phrases like 'You've got nothing to worry about', or 'You've got a 90 per cent chance that it's all right', for instance, which are so often said before surgery, are used more to protect the doctor from his own fears than to help the woman. Usually, they neither convince nor help her. Indeed, they may arouse even more anguish and fear in her because deep down she knows, even if she doesn't admit it to herself or anyone else, that she does have something real to worry about, otherwise why is she in this clinic having this examination or being sent for biopsy?

'They're frightened to tell you anything because they're afraid you're going to freak out on them,' one woman told me bitterly, and then added: 'You get more silence than anything. If you don't ask, they tell you nothing.'

The recent survey of 300 surgeons to which I have already referred several times reveals that they spend on average no more than ten minutes breaking the bad news, and only half those surveyed had the services of a nurse counsellor in their clinic. Even if a specialist nurse is not available, a basic sense of humanity would surely not permit the all too frequent situation where a woman is left to dress in silence, wander round the hospital making her appointments for further tests, and stumble out alone, her world collapsing around her.

'Some counselling, a cup of tea, an enquiry if they have transport, anyone at home, an assessment to see if they are fit to drive and some helpful literature to put the feet back on the ground should be automatic,' wrote an angry husband to Mrs Edwina Currie when she was Junior Minister for Health. He described his wife's treatment at the initial stage of diagnosis as 'bordering on the criminally negligent'.

Even those women who declare themselves happy with the medical care they received can usually recall some incident when they were met by an offhand or patronising response. Often they will excuse the doctor or nurse in question by saying that they realised how busy they were and that they could not be expected to deal with every little moan, or answer every question.

But can't they? Should it not be an integral part of good medical management that the patient's enquiries, fears and anxieties are dealt with as carefully as the physical symptoms are treated? Communication, compassion and concern are the three Cs that should never be left out of caring for cancer patients.

FEELINGS – DURING AND AFTER TREATMENT

The feelings you might expect to experience at this time don't come in an ordered sequence, nor will you necessarily feel all of them to the same degree of intensity. Some of them may not even be part of your personal experience, but what follows here are descriptions of emotions that women have talked about to me and to others. Some you will identify with strongly and others, perhaps, you will hardly understand, but that is because each one of us is a unique individual. Some feelings will be deeply personal to you; they well out of your spiritual depths and reflect your life, your experiences, your relationships and your private hopes and fears. Others are induced by the circumstances in which you now find yourself, your physical state and the quality of care that you are receiving. What matters is that whatever your feelings may be they belong to you, they are real, they are important and you must be allowed to feel free to express them and deal with them in the way that seems best to you.

Many women, when warned that they must expect a mastectomy, react with the words, 'How can I tell my husband?' They fear that he will reject them, repelled by a wife without a breast. Mothers are seized with dread that they may never live to see their children grow up. Single women fear that they will never again have a lover. Elderly women who may already have suffered the loss of their husband cannot conceive how they can survive this new blow on their own. Lonely women will feel utterly bereft and friendless. Even the woman who is lucky enough to be surrounded by a loving family and friends may now feel terribly alone and unwilling to confide in those who are closest to her because she feels she can't endure the pain and unhappiness they will be feeling for her.

These are all feelings related to other people, and they are very typical of how women perceive themselves; they are putting the feelings of those who are close to them first, and only later do they start thinking about themselves.

Anger may be one of the first direct emotions to hit them. 'Why me? What have I done to deserve this?' Young women, women who have been hoping to have babies, women who have looked after themselves and led principled lives, may feel outraged by what they regard as this unfair attack on them. Anger needs a target, someone to blame, and often the person nearest to hand is the doctor or nurse. Health professionals, under stress themselves, may react badly – either defensively or punitively – to the onslaught, and this can set up a vicious circle of abuse and hurt, followed by rejection and withdrawal. This is where the intervention of a trained counsellor can be invaluable if the doctor has the wisdom to recognise that he can't always handle every situation.

Anger can also be healthy. It can be a way of defusing a

situation which has developed into a state of unbearable tension; it can force a doctor or nurse to apologise and start the relationship anew on a better footing; it can spur a patient to fight her illness because she is determined to prove the prognosis wrong.

A brutal diagnosis can cause anger in a woman, but so can evasive language and behaviour which will make her increasingly suspicious that something sinister is being withheld from her. This is a bad start to her programme of treatment and it only becomes worse if the doctor continues to deflect her questions after she has been told she will lose her breast. Patients who want to discuss treatment options are sometimes made to feel that they are a nuisance and unreasonable in their demands. Even if a woman accepts that a mastectomy is necessary or indeed decides she would prefer it, as many women do, it is still important that she should be treated honestly.

Signing the consent form can be a particularly harrowing experience and should be handled with sensitivity and only after the doctor is sure the patient fully understands the implications. Regrettably, this important task is too often left to a junior doctor who is inexperienced and nervous and not even knowledgeable enough to answer properly any questions the woman might want to ask. It certainly shouldn't happen this way: 'The form was just pushed under my nose with the doctor saying "sign there" and it wasn't until I read it that I realised I had breast cancer. When I asked him, was it true? he just said, "You've got nothing to worry about." No explanation, nothing.'

After a mastectomy it continues to be very important for the doctor to be as honest and straightforward as possible. Euphemisms like 'we caught it on the turn' or 'we caught it in time before it became cancer' fool no one, least of all the woman who knows in her heart, even if she dare not say so aloud, that you don't lose a breast lightly. If the doctor has been overconfident beforehand that he is certain the lump will prove harmless and a woman then wakes up to find that she has had a mastectomy, this will, quite naturally, make her feel deeply deceived. She may react bitterly and angrily, or withdraw into silent depression. Many women have told me that despite their doctor's misplaced optimism, they always felt that the tumour would turn out to be malignant, and waking to find their worst fears confirmed didn't help them to come to terms with the situation. Hospital staff who refuse to recognise these absolutely natural reactions by maintaining a breezy, bracing manner with remarks like 'Buck up, dear, there are worse things in life than losing a breast' or, alternatively, take it personally when the patient's distress spills out in complaints, only intensify her misery.

(This barbaric procedure of doing a mastectomy immediately following a frozen section analysis of the tumour while the patient is on the operating table should have been outlawed by now. However, letters coming into the Breast Care and Mastectomy Association reveal that it is still happening in many hospitals up and down the country. There is more discussion about consent to this and other procedures in chapter 17.)

Many women need time to grieve for the lost breast: 'M said he would still love me with one breast. Before I went into hospital I said goodbye to myself. I stripped and stood in front of the mirror and looked at myself. To remember. After surgery, when the bandage had come off, I went into the bathroom, looked at myself and wept.' Not all women are able to look at their scar so soon, or they feel shamed and revolted by the disfigurement and believe that others who see it will feel likewise, so they hide away from their partner and their children.

Others are clawed by guilt. Why have they been struck by this terrible disease? What sin in their past life has singled them out for this dreadful punishment? It doesn't help if people close to them behave rather as if they felt the same. There is a dangerous tendency among a few amateur complementary health practitioners, and some doctors as well, to blame cancer patients for their illness. They have been eating the wrong food, thinking the wrong thoughts, leading a 'bad' life in some way, and this is why they are ill now. While it is possible that stress or repressed emotions may play some part in the appearance of breast cancer, no one can say with any certainty why or how this happens. As we shall see later, there are some cancers where there is a definite link to certain habits – smoking being the prime example – but this cannot be said of breast cancer. No one knows what causes it, and definitely no blame or guilt should be attached to any woman who contracts it, or indeed any other cancer. Victim-blaming is a negative and destructive activity.

COMMUNICATION

On the whole, women who are denied the truth or given roundabout answers or even contradictory information by different members of the health team end up by believing no one and nothing. They become angry and disinclined to accept the truth, even when it is finally offered to them. And if they have been lulled into a false sense of security – 'We've got it all out' – only later to find their hopes cruelly dashed – 'I'm afraid it's come back' – again, they will feel betrayed and angry. For instance, the woman who has not had an operation because her cancer was too advanced may have been told that 'it was not cancer but could turn into it unless treated with radiotherapy'. How is she going to feel when, inevitably, she discovers not only the grim truth but additionally that she has been lied to? One woman to whom something like this happened turned on the junior nurse whom she had befriended and attacked her bitterly for 'joining up with the rest of the bastards' – that is, her relatives and the doctors who had decided that she would not be able to bear hearing the truth of her condition. The woman died angry and unforgiving and the nurse, who was only doing what she was told – and very much against her will – is haunted by the memory.

Doctors do have a very difficult job, but it's even harder to be a patient. No one should pretend that communication is easy, particularly with cancer patients who have a life-threatening disease, but if this is a doctor's chosen speciality, then part of that work lies in establishing an honest and, as far as possible, co-operative partnership with each of their patients. The patient is not just a bunch of deviant cells or an organ exhibiting interesting symptoms. She is a person with needs, emotions and a life history beyond her hospital bed. This is a moment in her life when she feels deeply threatened and isolated. Her femininity, her relationships, even her life may be at stake. She wants to feel that she is still a person, a woman; certainly not a mere object of detached curiosity or someone who can be treated with less respect because she has suddenly become vulnerable and powerless in an impersonal institution.

Of course, not every woman does want to be told the facts, or at least not all at once. Some will say something like, 'Don't tell me the details. I don't want to know. I know you're doing the best you can. I leave it to you,' and if that is how an individual woman wants to cope with her illness, her wishes should be respected. This is a form of denial and it is probably being used to numb the mental pain, rather as we use drugs to control physical pain; it is a way of absorbing shock and winning time to deal with the crisis and adjust to a new reality. Some women may go further and deny categorically that they have ever had cancer. Again, this is their way of coping, and it would be most unwise to try and make them 'face the facts', as it were. Deep down, whatever people may say, they usually do guess the truth, and even accept it tacitly, but they may not want to talk about it – at least, not for the time being.

But most women do want to know what is wrong with them, even if they are afraid to ask directly. A doctor has to learn to tune in to unspoken questions and to listen for unspoken answers, and some are much better at this than others. When the questions are asked they should be answered as frankly as possible and not in the unnerving manner described by one woman, whose surgeon always avoided direct contact. Instead he would stand at the foot of her bed 'muttering' to the sister while glancing from time to time in her direction.

'What they don't realise', she said, 'is that it's not what you know which upsets you but what you don't know.' A simple, obvious truth, it would seem – one so often repeated by cancer patients, yet so often disregarded by doctors. Physical contact is also very reassuring – a hug, holding hands, making eye contact, talking *to* not *at* the patient – are all small but significant ways of acknowledging a common humanity. The doctor who can do this with genuine warmth confirms the dignity of his patient and certainly doesn't lose any of his own in the process.

CARING

An inspiring book, *Love, Medicine and Miracles*, written by Bernie Siegel, an American cancer surgeon, shows what a difference an open mind and a warm heart can make. He was on the point of giving up cancer surgery, and looking for another career because he felt he couldn't take the stress any longer, when a cancer patient showed him how he could transform his own life and improve the quality of life for many of his patients simply by rethinking his attitudes and changing his approach. So he stepped out from behind his desk, asked his patients to call him Bernie, shaved his head so that he could identify with their hair loss and 'committed the physician's cardinal sin: [he] got involved with [his] patients'. Of course he didn't stop there, and his account of how he works with his patients is totally riveting.

He pays glowing tribute to a certain type of patient he calls the Exceptional Patient, who in the British context would no doubt be dubbed by many doctors as 'neurotic' or 'a nuisance' or 'a troublemaker' – in short, this is the patient who refuses to lie down and die. Exceptional Patients refuse to be passive and 'good'. They see themselves as survivors, not victims. They question everything, they are uninhibited about expressing their emotions – including the less socially acceptable ones like hostility, anger and distress – and they demand to be told as much as possible about their illness. They care about themselves. They want to retain control, and they are determined to beat their disease. Even if it gets them in the end (and after all, we do all have to die of something) they will go out like 'a tired lion not a frightened lamb', as a wife wrote about her husband.

Dr Stephen Greer, a psychologist at the Marsden Hospital who has done much pioneering research with breast cancer patients, has identified this same group as the ones with 'fighting spirit'. His follow-up studies show that these women tend to survive quite remarkably longer than more negative types like the 'helpless/hopeless' or the quiet stoics who give up because they think that nothing more can be done or quite simply take a fatalistic view that their time is up. There is a fourth, more ambivalent group, the 'deniers' described earlier, who turn their denial into a form of 'positive avoidance'. These women firmly put their illness behind them and behave as if it had never happened. They don't want to talk about it and they don't seek any help or sympathy. Women who behave like this also tend to survive longer.

Dr Greer is currently running a therapy programme for patients he has identified as suffering from severe psychological distress to try to help them overcome their problems and develop appropriate coping strategies. For instance, he will encourage them to discuss their treatment options with their doctors and he will also help them, in conjunction with their partner, to do some 'reality-testing'.

A typical example is the woman who feels that her mastectomy has deprived her of sexual attraction. Her husband, or partner, won't want her any more. Her friends are rejecting her. She feels stigmatised and isolated. Some of these perceptions may be true, but not all. For a start, has she asked her partner what he thinks? More often than not she will be surprised and reassured to find that he does not think like that at all but he does need some help too, to make the first approaches. He is probably just as frightened of cancer as she is, or he may be so concerned not to say the wrong thing and upset his wife further that he says nothing, thus confirming her feelings of rejection.

Even the strongest cancer survivor will have negative feelings many times during her treatment, and later, as she comes to terms with the realisation that cancer, even if it leaves your body, never completely leaves your mind. Now as never before, even if you have previously participated in the experience of death with a relative or friend, you are touched by a sense of your own mortality. Some people describe this as a transforming experience. They feel something verging on euphoria as they sense that they have been brushed by death and survived. One woman describes the whole process as 'a spiritual adventure' which is still going on many years later. She said that after the operation she felt happier than she had done for a long time. Life seemed wonderfully sweet and precious; the whole world was very beautiful and she was immensely glad to be in it. She was asked to talk to the nurses five days after her mastectomy and believes that she gave them a manic lecture about life seen through her rose-tinted spectacles. Six months later a depression set in which took a year to lift.

This kind of emotional rollercoastering is perfectly understandable. You are not going mad if you feel besieged by conflicting emotions, or just so terribly low that you wonder whether you will every feel 'normal' again. Cancer is a unique experience for each person who has it. Some people say they feel almost grateful for having gone through it, despite the suffering, because it has given them a new, more meaningful perspective on life. They have reassessed their priorities, their important relationships have become much deeper and closer, and they now live each day as it comes. Others may have more difficulty in finding a positive way forward, at least to begin with, and need help. No one should think herself inadequate for feeling like this, but it is important to find the help and information that are right for you.

[11]

Help is there

This chapter suggests other people who might be able to help you and tells you where good practical advice and information are available. It also contains some exercises and other ideas for recovering your physical fitness as quickly as possible.

SOMEONE TO TALK TO . . .

The *nurse counsellor* is a senior oncology nurse who will have had considerable experience of taking care of cancer patients before training as a counsellor. She will also have been trained to fit prostheses (breast forms), so she brings a combination of interpersonal and specialised practical skills to her job and, since she has chosen to do this work and has been carefully selected for it, she is likely to be rather a special person in herself: mature and sympathetic – in fact, the ideal friend.

The Forrest Report emphasises how important it is to have one of these nurses in every screening clinic. Here her role is to be on hand from the moment a woman arrives for her appointment, tell her about the procedures and answer any questions she may have. If the woman is recalled for any reason, the nurse counsellor will be there to reassure her and give her further information. The screening centres are run fairly autonomously within each health region, so it's not possible to say precisely what will happen when and in what sequence. If, however, the woman is referred to an assessment centre in the nearest hospital for further testing, it is to be hoped that the set-up is organised in such a way that the same nurse counsellor is present when she attends this centre or clinic, because it is now that she has a very important role to play.

She will be there to explain how the tests are done, and for what purpose. She can accompany the woman to her various appointments and hold her hand, literally as well as figuratively, and be there to comfort and support her if the doctor has to give her a diagnosis of cancer. She is the calm, steady friend most of us would like to be able to turn to in bad times, and her presence is all the more helpful very often just because she is *not* really a friend but a well-trained professional who draws on a wealth of experience and caring skills.

She will spend as much or as little time with her clients as they wish. Some women will want to unburden themselves about many problems, and she will be there to listen in a non-directive way. Others will decide they need very little of her time, perhaps just some practical information about exercises or a prosthesis. The nurse counsellor will be sensitive to these different needs and never feel hurt or rebuffed because someone has said she doesn't want to talk to her. In many ways the role of a nurse counsellor is more negatively than positively orientated. For instance, it's not her job to tell women what they should do, or try to solve their personal problems for them, or prevent them from being upset. This is how one experienced counsellor has defined her role: 'I'm there to help people help themselves, to enable them to reach greater self-understanding and mobilise their own coping abilities.'

One of the very important things a nurse counsellor can do is to help a woman think through her various treatment options. To do this well, she needs to give the woman plenty of information, written as well as verbal, and plenty of space to think and talk about the implications of her decision. Before the woman comes into hospital for her treatment she will tell her the order of events and what she will feel like when she comes round from the anaesthetic if she has had surgery – for instance, that it is normal to feel numbness followed by a sense of constriction if it has been a mastectomy – and she will explain the need for drainage tubes and other post-operative procedures.

Soon after the woman has had her operation, the nurse counsellor will be at her bedside. Although she does not do any direct nursing herself, she closely follows the patient's recovery. She discusses prostheses and bras with her, shows her models and gives her a lightly fitting one which she can wear for the first few weeks while the scar heals. She helps the patient with her exercises and, of course, is there to be a sympathetic listener about any problems she may have, or fears are waiting for her at home.

The nurse counsellor does not say goodbye to her client when she leaves the hospital. By now she will have come to know the woman's partner, members of her family, or whoever else is especially close to her. If she is a woman on her own, perhaps rather lonely, the nurse counsellor can take the place of the missing friend. When the patient goes home she continues to be available to her at the end of a telephone line, or to make a home visit if that is what the patient would prefer.

At its most complete, this is a wonderful service to offer women with breast cancer. Unfortunately, some doctors are not convinced about the merits of counselling; they tend to think of it as something 'soft', potentially dangerous in 'the wrong hands' – i.e. the patient may be upset or become too demanding – so they are not prepared to negotiate for the necessary funding to staff this post. These same doctors are unlikely to agree with Bernie Siegel's view (described in the last chapter) that these are actually healthy reactions and to be preferred to the passive 'good patient' syndrome. There are even some doctors who regard any information coming from outside their radius of control with suspicion, so that they ban even quite innocuous but useful leaflets from voluntary organisations from their wards. Of course an untrained, overenthusiastic amateur counsellor *is* a liability and can do more harm than good, but this is not the job description of a nurse counsellor. Interestingly – and apart from the rare sister who fears that 'her' patients are being usurped – ward nurses tend to feel quite differently from doctors. They appreciate that the nurse counsellor, with her specialist skills, can fill in the gaps for which they have neither the knowledge nor the time. Not all women will want to be counselled and they can say so, should the service be offered to them, but generally speaking it is reasonable to believe that there are more women up and down the country who are left floundering and unhappy for lack of the most basic information and little, if any, moral and emotional support.

The volunteer is a woman who has had breast surgery herself and is prepared to talk to another woman who is about to have, or has just been through, a similar experience. The Breast Care and Mastectomy Association (BCMA) is the main channel through which these volunteers operate. This organisation was set up in 1971 by Betty Westgate, who had been through the lonely experience of mastectomy in the days when absolutely no information or help of any kind was given out to women. She herself received her diagnosis over the telephone. Betty realised that she was comparatively fortunate since she had a loving husband and family waiting for her at home, unlike many women who, she knew, were leaving the cocooned atmosphere of the hospital ward to return to lives of lonely desperation and had no one to whom they could turn.

You don't need any special qualifications to be a volunteer: just kindness, common sense and a reasonable amount of understanding and patience. You must also have had your own treatment at least two years earlier, because it is important that you should not obtrude any lingering anxieties of your own into someone else's experience. Some volunteers may have done a short course in counselling, but mostly they are sympathetic women who remember what it felt like for them and would like to help someone else through her bad patches. They will listen and empathise but they are pledged not to offer any amateur psychologising nor pseudo-medical advice. Basically, what they are giving is practical information – like which is the best local shop for suitable underwear, or where it is possible to buy a better prosthesis. They also offer the reassurance and understanding that only someone who has been through the same sort of experience can give. They don't encourage self-pity, but if a caller does seem very upset and plainly in need of professional help they will refer her back to their regional organiser, who will put her in touch with an appropriate person.

If you have had breast surgery and reading this makes you feel you would like to be a volunteer, write to the BCMA at its London headquarters (see Resources), which will refer you to your nearest organiser. This woman will interview you before adding you to her local register of names. She tries to match caller and volunteer as closely as possible in terms of age, marital status and social circumstances, thus making it easier to strike a common bond.

The BCMA is run by women, several of whom have had breast cancer themselves. In addition to answering queries by letter and on the telephone, they send out very good and regularly updated free leaflets to help women with practical problems after surgery. They also have an excellent video featuring several of their volunteers exchanging tips and experiences about buying clothes. Visitors to their offices can look through new lines of swimwear, bras and prostheses.

BACUP Cancer Information Service is a nationwide free telephone service, answered by trained cancer nurses who can help you with most queries you may have. Anything they don't know how to answer they will refer back to one of their medical advisers. They can also put you in touch with your nearest support group and send you free information booklets (see Resources).

Support groups are often set up on a fairly informal basis
by someone who has had breast cancer and feels she would
like to share her experiences and help other women in the
same situation. Occasionally they may be organised by a
sympathetic doctor or nurse. Not everyone is attracted by the
idea of joining a group where the common bond is cancer,
but for others the relief of being able to relax among people
who really do understand their problems, because they have
had them too, can be marvellously therapeutic.

REACH TO RECOVERY – IN HOSPITAL

Soon after the operation you will be encouraged to start
getting up and moving around, walking to the toilet and
sitting in a chair. Apart from the awkwardness of having to
carry with you drainage tubes which are fixed inside your
stitches to draw off excess fluid, you may find that the arm
on the operation side is uncomfortable if you let it hang
down. You may also feel thrown off balance.

'Breasts are heavier than you think,' one medium-sized
woman pointed out to me, and said that it had surprised her
how long it took to adjust to this shift in weight. If you have
a big bosom this can be a real problem but it is important to
get it right as soon as possible, otherwise your posture
changes, resulting in muscular aches and pains elsewhere in
your body – a complication you can well do without.

Here are a couple of simple suggestions originated by the
American Reach to Recovery organisation, to cope with these
difficulties.

1 Arm support

Ask the nurse or one of your visitors to roll up a towel or a
strip of foam rubber into a sausage about eighteen inches
long and six inches thick, which she then ties with a two-inch
bandage in three places. Each length of bandage should be
long enough to go diagonally across your chest and back and

tie round your neck on your unaffected side. The roll is thus held against your body under your armpit, and you can rest your aching arm on it. You will probably find it useful at home as well for the first few weeks until your arm has fully recovered.

2 Breast support

To make this you need a piece of soft, easily draped material about one-and-a-quarter yards square, some large safety pins and a small firm pad of folded material roughly four inches square.

The nurse must help you by folding the material into a triangle; then, placing your breast comfortably into the middle of the triangle, she takes a slightly longer end under your breast and arm, round up your back and over your shoulder to meet the shorter end just above your breast. Rather than tie the sling, which causes pressure because of the weight of your breast, she should fold the two ends neatly and pin them together on top of the small pad. To give the sling a cup shape which will hold your breast firmly, she pins two more safety pins in the appropriate places to make the darts. You may find this sling even more useful to wear at home when you are doing the housework and until you have had your permanent prosthesis fitted, which will restore your balance.

If your operation has been either a simple or a modified radical your scar will run neatly across your chest in a transverse line well below any low-necked dress or swimsuit that you might wish to wear later on. Until the time comes to take out your stitches, your wound will be dressed regularly. Although this sounds terribly hard, it may help you in the long run if you can try looking downwards when the nurse does this so as to get used to the flatness. If you find this impossible, don't worry. Now is not the time to force yourself over too many hurdles, and many women find this a particularly daunting one. Sometime, though, you will probably have to look at yourself in a mirror and it may be easier to do it quietly on your own in the hospital, so that you can work through some of your grieving before you return to your family.

As soon as you begin to feel better in yourself, you should be doing some gentle exercising under instruction from the physiotherapist to mobilise your arm on the operation side. This is going to be painful at the beginning, but it is worth pushing yourself because the sooner you start exercising your stiff muscles, the less likelihood there is that they will shrink from lack of use, making it more difficult for you to use your arm freely later on. If nothing has been prescribed for you after the first few days, make a point of asking why. Some doctors are much more punctilious than others about this aspect of treatment but the old idea that the arm should be kept immobile for a fortnight has been superseded, unless for some particular reason your operation requires it. While your stitches are still in you must obviously not be too energetic, but the physiotherapist will guide you in this.

3 Arm exercises (to be continued at home)

These should be done in the following order and on the principle of a little at a time. Never strain yourself, but make a point of reaching a little further and a little longer each time you do them. Remember that it is always the arm on your operation side which is being exercised. Ask for your doctor's advice before you start.

(1) HAIR BRUSHING

Prop your arm on a pile of books placed on your dressing-table. Sit straight, hold your head up and start brushing one side of your head. Gradually work all the way round, possibly at different times until you are able to brush all your hair.

(II) NEWSPAPER CRUMPLING

Place a pile of separated newspaper pages on a table and rest your arm on it from elbow to wrist. Crumple the pages completely, one by one. Squeezing a soft rubber ball in your hand, which you can do at any time of day (in a standing position) has the same effect of strengthening the hand and arm muscles.

(III) WALKING UP THE WALL

Stand with feet apart (flat shoes or barefoot) facing the wall, with your forehead resting against it. Gradually reach upwards, pressing the wall lightly with your hands. Do this slowly and often, but don't overtax yourself. Eventually you will be able to reach right above your head with your arms straight.

(IV) ROPE SWINGING

Tie a length of rope round a door handle. Stand or sit at right angles to it, holding the other hand lightly but firmly in your affected hand. Start swinging it gently in small circles, gradually making them bigger as your arm becomes more flexible.

As you get more practised you can devise other exercises for yourself, based on the same reaching principle, but do remember not to overdo it. There are also several household chores which use the same muscles, like hanging up the washing, reaching up to a top shelf or cleaning the windows. What you must avoid is lifting anything heavy, pushing or pulling. Typing and knitting are also good exercises.

CHOOSING A PROSTHESIS

If you are lucky you will have a nurse counsellor to help you with this. There are at least fifteen types available on the

NHS, and of course many more if you are willing to pay for one in a specialist shop. Unfortunately, many hospitals are extremely offhand about the whole business, offering only a very limited range and no real advice about how to wear a prosthesis. Some seem to be unaware that the days of birdseed bags and inert shapeless lumps which have a disconcerting habit of dropping out of the bra when a woman bends over are long since gone. Usually the person fitting breast prostheses is the surgical appliance officer, who is sometimes a man. He may try to be sensitive and discreet, but it's hard to imagine a more off-putting situation for a women who is struggling to adjust to her disfigurement than to have a non-medical male stranger fitting her with something so intimate and personal to her.

The BCMA have done their own researches and are horrified by the indifference, verging on callousness, that so many nurses and doctors show towards this important aspect of rehabilitation. A recent survey published in the *Nursing Mirror*[1] revealed that women were pitifully uninformed when they went for their first fitting and that 'there is no consistent way in which the patients are informed of the provision of prostheses. It is not clear whose responsibility it is to tell them' – from which one can assume that probably no one does.

Don't suffer in silence. If you encounter any problems in this area, telephone the BCMA, who will send you a comprehensive lists of stockists, or you can visit their own offices, where they keep a wide range of the latest prostheses. It is important to know that this choice is available because each woman is different in shape and taste: some, for instance, would like the prosthesis to be as like a real breast as possible, including a nipple, so that they can continue to wear tight-fitting jumpers and blouses; others are more concerned just to have the correct weight and the fullness matching their other breast so that they can feel comfortable and look as they always have done. The women at the BCMA are experienced and sympathetic, as are the specially trained mastectomy fitters to be found in certain high-street stores and specialist shops.

PRECAUTIONS

Lymphoedema (heavy arm) is a troublesome complication which sometimes arises after radiotherapy or radical surgery when the lymph glands have been removed. The arm swells and can become very painful. To be on the safe side:

1 Always offer your unaffected arm for vaccination, injections, blood sampling or blood pressure testing.

2 Protect your hand and arm against cuts, burns and scrapes.

3 Wear loose-fitting gloves for household chores and gardening.

4 Protect your arm against sunburn.

5 Wear a thimble for sewing.

6 Use an electric razor for under-arm shaving.

7 Avoid carrying heavy shopping bags or suitcases with your affected arm.

8 Keep your arm supported as much as possible. At night you can sleep with it on a pillow, holding it above your head. At least you can start off with it in that position.

If you develop an infection, however slight, see your doctor immediately, as prompt action could spare you considerable and sometimes lasting discomfort. Sometimes lymphoedema cannot be prevented, in which case you must see your doctor. There are also ways you can help yourself, but get your doctor's agreement first. Crepe bandaging at night or wearing an elastic sleeve are two methods, the aim being to support, not constrict. It is also possible to reduce the swelling by using a mechanical pump and sleeve, but you should do this only on medical advice.

REACH FOR RECOVERY – AT HOME

Even though it's good to be home with your family and sleeping in your own bed, there may be moments when you miss the protective warmth and camaraderie of the hospital ward. More time spent on your own also means more time thinking about your problems. Physically you will tire easily, especially if you are having radiotherapy or chemotherapy, and temporary handicaps caused by your stiff muscles may assume undue proportions. If you have a job it is a good idea to go back to it as soon as you feel strong enough, because the stimulus provided by your work and colleagues will help you to forget your own problems. The mother with young children will also be distracted by the constant attention she must give to them, but it may be harder for the woman who is usually alone at home during the day.

Whoever you are, you probably won't want to fling yourself immediately into a mad social whirl but equally, don't shrink away from your friends or usual activities. Many people will want to help but they will feel nervous about intruding, so sometimes you will have to take the initiative. Ease yourself back into your old life. It hasn't come to a full stop because of your illness, but there has been a pause and it has changed.

PART TWO

Other cancers affecting women

[12]

The one we needn't have

AN IMMORAL TALE

Every year around 2,000 women in this country die of cervical cancer. Almost every one of these deaths is a special tragedy, because it should never have happened. Two-thirds of them, mostly older women, will never have had a cervical smear. Others may have come for a smear too late, and some will have died because even though they did all the right things, 'the system' failed them.

Cancer of the cervix is possibly the only cancer in our present state of knowledge that is truly preventable. With rare exceptions its existence can be predicted and averted many years before it will develop into a full-blown malignancy; the test for this is simple, painless and cheap. The 'pap' smear was invented more than sixty years ago by Dr George Papanicolaou, a Greek doctor working in America, and involves no more than scraping a few cells off the cervix and investigating them under a microscope. Should any abnormal changes be detected, requiring treatment, there are now several procedures to choose from, all of them quick, relatively painless, devoid of serious side-effects and cost-effective.

We have had a cervical screening programme in Britain since 1966 but in the last decade the mortality rate has declined by only 14 per cent, a figure which compares badly with other countries. Over the same period, the incidence of positive smears as a proportion of all smears taken has increased by 50

per cent and there has been a particularly worrying increase
among women in their twenties and thirties.

When things go wrong it is always tempting to look for
scapegoats and lay the blame elsewhere. Doctors say women
are not coming forward; women say they are often inad-
equately informed or are discouraged from coming back
because of the way they have been treated; everyone (with
some justice) blames a disorganised service with no uniform
method of call and recall, frequent breakdowns of communication between the various professional groups, and a disastrous incidence of bureaucratic muddles.

There is also an unappealing whiff of moral censure
hanging around the whole topic. Sex and the cervix: everyone
knows just enough to know that they are closely linked, and
it is not uncommon to suggest that too much of the one
causes problems for the other. Is it surprising, therefore, that
elderly women who have been faithfully married to a single
partner all their lives, or women who have been widowed or
single for years, can't see what it's got to do with them? Or
that younger women, upset by intrusive and censorious
questioning about their sex lives and offended by a punitive
attitude which doesn't have to be verbally expressed to make
itself felt, refuse to return for repeat smears or follow-up?

The truth is that any woman who has had sexual intercourse at any time is at risk of cervical cancer. It used to be
said that virgins and nuns were exempt, but even this sacred
axiom has been questioned recently in an only half-joking
request for 'scientific continence' by that scourge of the
medical establishment, Dr Petr Skrabanek.[1] His researches
reveal that there are extremely rare but documented cases of
virginal women who have developed cervical cancer – a fact
which merely goes to show that cancer of the cervix, like the
other 200-plus varieties of this disease, is complex and
multifactorial in origin.

The present situation is that there are many suspects lined
up for ongoing investigation, but no one single factor which
can be conclusively proved to cause cervical cancer. This

being so, until we have hard facts in favour of one or more of them – and it seems highly likely that they interact upon each other – it is much more constructive to work along the guidelines thrown up by the existing evidence and identify high-risk groups. There is no moralising attached to this: all it means is that something in their circumstances, their state of health or certain aspects of their lifestyle may render them more vulnerable to the possibility of developing a *predisposition* to cervical cancer. That's all – not the cancer itself, which can be latent for as long as fifteen to twenty years. Nevertheless, many women who develop abnormal smears don't conform to any of the high-risk classifications – which emphasises how important it is that no woman ever passes up her appointment for a smear.

The real moral of this tale must by now be clear. Due to some quite remarkable medical advances, we have the means to prevent this cancer. We can actually stop it before it starts, and this wonderful facility should be known and available to everyone. One of the prime principles behind offering a screening service is that you can follow it up with the necessary treatments as and when they are required. It is, therefore, a scandalous and immoral state of affairs that many women are still not being screened for cervical cancer, perhaps for lack of adequate education or because they have been frightened off, while others are coming forward but may be kept waiting for months before they receive the treatment they need, and sometimes don't even get it then.

REASONS FOR HAVING A SMEAR TEST

You started an active sexual life more than two years ago;

You are between twenty and sixty-five and are or have been sexually active.

The current official recommendation is that smears should be taken every five years, but many doctors would prefer the interval to be reduced to three. Women at special risk are anyway now asked to present themselves more often; ideally at yearly intervals and, of course, even more frequently if they have an 'abnormal' smear which needs to be checked. However, since there is also considerable concern about the large numbers of women who are missing the screening net altogether, the policy-makers at the Department of Health feel that immediate efforts should concentrate on improving health education and making the service more 'user-friendly' so that women will feel less reluctant to take up the invitation.

It is a pity that with the present impetus to encourage all eligible women to come forward for breast screening, the two services cannot be combined as a matter of course under one roof, but it seems to be a case of a house divided against itself. One part of the medical establishment – that concerned with breast cancer – is so horrified by the muddling through it has seen in the cervical screening programme that it is determined to steer well clear of any involvement. Whether this will ultimately prove to be in the best interests of women is another matter; meanwhile, we have to take advantage of what is offered.

WHERE TO GO FOR A SMEAR

Your GP will be able to do it for you, but if you are already going to a family planning clinic or a well woman clinic you may prefer it to be done there. A smear is always taken if you are pregnant.

Some GPs will ask their patients if they have had a smear recently and operate their own system of call and recall, but as things are at the moment most women have to remember to make their own appointments. This is very important, so try and devise some way of reminding yourself. Arrange for it to be as close to the middle of your cycle as you can manage because the smear should be taken when the cervix is free of menstrual flow.

All health authorities have now installed computerised call and recall systems, and between now and 1993 they aim to have invited for screening all women between twenty and sixty-four (about thirteen million). These systems, efficiently operated, should ensure that every woman is entered on the computer when she has her first smear and is automatically reminded when she should come again. But more than this is necessary to make the system work really well: laboratories must report results more rapidly, preferably within a month; abnormal smears must always be followed up. And there must be adequate facilities for prompt and appropriate treatment when necessary.

HOW A SMEAR IS TAKEN

Having a smear taken involves a brief internal examination. You lie on a couch and a speculum is inserted to open your vagina in order to inspect your cervix, which is at the top of the vagina. The cervix is the neck of the uterus (womb); it has a central hole called the os (cervical canal) through which menstrual blood is passed every month. The os is also the gateway to sperm entering the uterus and ultimately, if conception has taken place, it expands to allow the baby to leave the uterus, enter the birth canal (vagina) and be born.

Women who use tampons or a diaphragm (cap) for contraception will be used to feeling their cervix, which is a bit like a nose – blobby and mobile. You can in fact look at your own cervix with the aid of a speculum, mirror and light or torch. Some doctors will help a woman to do this during an examination, or you can do it for yourself at home.

To take the smear the doctor or nurse uses a spatula, made of wood or plastic, and gently scrapes a few cells off the cervix. This does not hurt but you may feel tense and nervous, especially if it is the first time. Most doctors are aware of this and will encourage you to relax. Some doctors are now using a cytobrush, which looks a bit like a tiny pipe cleaner, because they can insert it a little higher inside the os, into what is called the endocervix, and collect more cells. This is not painful but it sometimes causes a bit of spotting afterwards.

The area from which the cells have been taken just around and inside the os is called the transformation zone because it is here that two different sorts of cells meet: the squamous cells, forming the external surface of the cervix, and the columnar endometrial cells, which constitute the internal lining (endometrium) of your uterus. It is these cells that are examined under the microscope by a cytologist to see if there are any abnormal changes in their structure.

You may be told by the doctor that you will be contacted only if your smear is positive, or a repeat smear is considered necessary, possibly for some technical reason like the cytologist not having enough cells for analysis. Mistakes with tragic consequences have happened in the past when women with positive smears were not informed, so don't accept this if it makes you feel uneasy. Do not hesitate to ring the surgery for confirmation of the result and if it is negative, which means there is nothing wrong, the receptionist can give you the information over the telephone. This ensures that your name has not been overlooked.

AN ABNORMAL (POSITIVE) SMEAR DOES NOT MEAN CANCER

It means that something is causing the cells to change in their overall size or appearance, or is increasing the size of the cell nucleus. The change could be due to an infection or could be an indication that these changes, if left unchecked, might eventually become a cancer. If an infection is diagnosed it can usually be treated with antibiotics or cream of some sort. You will then be called back for another smear to check that the infection has cleared and that the cells are now normal.

The cells may show signs of being infected with a genital wart virus known as human papilloma virus (HPV); and this is called koilocytosis. Since it is thought that certain strains of this virus (HPV 16 and 18) could cause pre-cancerous changes in the cells, this is always an indication for further examination as well as treatment, but it is worth knowing that many women who have this infection never develop anything more sinister.

Any abnormal changes in cell structure are called *dysplasia* (bad shape) or *dyskariosis* (bad nucleus). According to the degree of change noted, they are graded as mild, moderate or severe. Very often the mild or moderate dysplasias return to normal in a few months' time. Both cervical abnormalities and cervical cancer are undoubtedly on the increase among younger women, but whether they also progress more rapidly than in older women is open to question. Although there have been some publications suggesting this, it has not been confirmed by any of the large-scale studies. Any woman presenting with an abnormal smear will be asked to come back for a further smear after three to six months. If it still proves abnormal, she should be referred to a colposcopy clinic for further examination.

There is a new technique called cervicography, which involves taking a photograph of the cervix at the same time as the smear. It is simple and easy to do and is a useful back-up to the smear because it reduces the rate of false negative smears to practically zero. It is difficult to assess the true rate of false negatives – estimates veer wildly from 10 to 50 per cent – but much depends on the standard of cytology. Probably a fair estimate in this country is about 15 per cent. Before taking the photograph, called a cervigram, the doctor or nurse wipes the cervix with a weak vinegar solution which makes any abnormal areas show up white. One picture is enough and it is sent for assessment to a gynaecologist. Although this method is widely used in the United States it is still undergoing trials in this country, so it is available only in a few clinics.

POSITIVE SMEAR, POSITIVE ACTION – INVESTIGATION

A positive smear result means you must have a more detailed examination at a colposcopy clinic. Your doctor will make an appointment, but do make sure it is not fixed at a time when you are expecting your period. The colposcopy clinic is usually run by a gynaecologist with nurses and, preferably, a counsellor, who does not need to be medically trained. She is, though, an important member of the team because, not unnaturally, this is an emotionally fraught time for most women.

For a start you may feel embarrassed by the way the colposcopic examination has to be done. No one can pretend that this is anything but an ungainly and undignified procedure, but in most clinics everyone is sympathetic and will do their best to put you at your ease. In some you can even watch your own examination on a video. You may also be very worried about the diagnosis and this will make you tense and rigid, which doesn't help when you are being examined. Some doctors encourage women to bring their partner or a close friend, but even if you prefer to go through this on your own, a nurse or counsellor will be there to explain what is going on. Try to relax as much as possible by deep breathing.

First, the nurse will ask you to remove your pants and tights. It is sensible to wear a full skirt, which you can keep on, rather than trousers, which will obviously have to come off. She will then help you into a special chair which is adjustable to different angles and heights, rather like a dentist's chair. You hook your legs over supports on either side so that they flop apart, enabling the doctor to insert the speculum to open your vagina. Then the colposcope is wheeled into position. This is a microscope on a stand, which has a magnifying lens and a light, enabling the doctor to look through it at the cervix. The cervix will be washed with a weak vinegar solution, in the same way as for a cervigram and for the same reason. Sometimes iodine is also used because it is better at showing up abnormal areas, particularly if the doctor wants to take a biopsy. This involves cutting minute pieces of tissue, no larger than a pinhead, from the cervix. This is called a punch biopsy and it may cause a brief sharp pain, but it can be avoided if the doctor guides you to cough at the exact moment the biopsy is taken. You may have slight bleeding afterwards and a feeling like a period pain, but this won't last long and some women feel nothing at all.

The examination is over, and it is unlikely to have taken more than ten minutes. Although by now the doctor will have a pretty good idea of your condition, he or she will want to wait for the biopsy results before making a definitive diagnosis and deciding on treatment. Whereas the cytologist bases the analysis of the smear on the appearance of the cells, the histopathologist at the laboratory grades the biopsy according to how deeply the abnormal cells have penetrated into the cervical structure.

CIN is an abbreviation for Cervical Intraepithelial Neoplasia which, translated into English, means a change in the superficial cell structure of the cervix. CIN I is mild dysplasia, CIN II is moderate dysplasia and CIN III is severe dysplasia. All stages of CIN indicate superficial changes only, but while a short-term watch-and-wait policy may be in order for CIN I and CIN II, CIN III must always be treated immediately. CIN III does *not* mean you have cancer, but it does indicate that the abnormal cells have gone further into the cervix towards what is called the basement membrane. This band of tissue separates the cervical tissue from the deeper connective tissue in the body and it is essential to eradicate the abnormal pre-cancerous cells before they penetrate the basement membrane and turn into micro-invasive cancer.

POSITIVE SMEAR, POSITIVE ACTION – TREATMENT

There are five main treatments for CIN III lesions, three of which can be done in the colposcopy clinic. The woman lies or sits back on the colposcopy couch in the lithotomy position, as described above for investigation. Usually one treatment session is sufficient to remove the problem and there are relatively few after-effects apart, possibly, from some period-like cramps for a short while and some light bleeding or discharge as the wound heals. You will be asked not to wear tampons for a month to six weeks and also, during the same period, to abstain from making love involving vaginal penetration. This is to allow the cervix a chance to heal. When the scab comes off the cervix, be prepared for some quite heavy bleeding and if it persists, telephone the colposcopy clinic or hospital clinic where you had the treatment. They will give you an emergency appointment to deal with the situation, which is not serious but can be alarming. It is also most important that you keep your follow-up appointments — usually made at three-monthly, six-monthly and finally yearly intervals — when your cervix will be examined with the colposcope and a smear taken to make sure that all has returned to normal.

OUTPATIENT TREATMENTS

Cryotherapy (cryocautery) destroys abnormal cells by freezing them. An instrument called a cryoprobe is inserted into the vagina and fitted over the cervix, through which a gas such as nitrous oxide is pumped at high speed and very low temperature. The actual freezing is done in two short sessions, usually about three minutes each with a five-minute break in between. You will probably feel a dull pelvic pain, like an early period pain, which will wear off quite quickly afterwards but can be helped with a mild painkiller. This is regarded as a very successful treatment, particularly for CIN I and II, but it may not be suitable for CIN III. It does cause a watery discharge which may last for a fortnight and some external scarring of the cervix which will have no effect on your sex life, fertility or childbearing.

Cold coagulation is a similar treatment but uses a probe heated to a high temperature, bearable without anaesthetic, to destroy the abnormal cells. (It is called 'cold' because it is much colder than the extreme heat used with electrodiathermy, described below.) It is similar in after-effects and results to cryocautery.

Laser therapy is the use of a high-energy beam of light to vaporise tissue; it literally burns it out of existence. This is regarded as the best treatment for CIN III because of its accuracy and ability to penetrate tissue, but it does require special training for the doctor and the equipment is much more expensive than for the other treatments, which is one reason why you may not always be offered it. The laser is attached to a colposcope, which enables the doctor to map out the cervical area to be treated and train the beam very directly on to it. It leaves no scars on the cervix, and the rate of success after one treatment only is well over 90 per cent. It does, however, cause quite severe pain to some women. We all vary considerably as to what we can tolerate, but there is no reason why women should suffer unnecessarily.[2] Many doctors will do this treatment with a local anaesthetic, as for a dental filling, and put some anaesthetic cream on the cervix afterwards. It is important not to move during the treatment, which lasts about ten minutes, so if you are feeling extremely tense and nervous about the procedure it can be done under general anaesthetic. Alternatively you could ask for your partner or a close friend to sit with you and hold your hand throughout.

TREATMENTS REQUIRING GENERAL ANAESTHETIC

Electrodiathermy uses very high temperatures to burn away cervical tissue, and is as effective as laser therapy. However, it is painful, so it has to be done under a light general anaesthetic. This can be done on a day-patient basis. You come in, having fasted several hours beforehand, the treatment is carried out, and you rest for a while afterwards. You may feel a bit sick and have period-like pains, so it is advisable to ask a friend or relative to take you home.

Cone biopsy involves removing a segment of the cervix containing abnormal cells. Before colposcopy it used to be both the method of diagnosis for CIN grading and the only treatment for all abnormal smears. Now it is used only in these circumstances:

> part of the abnormal area extends high up the cervical canal and cannot be seen on the colposcope (most usual reason);
>
> the doctor suspects that the abnormal cells may have spread through the basement membrane;
>
> persistent abnormal smears, though nothing can be seen on the colposcope;
>
> the doctor has no access to a colposcopy clinic.

A cone biopsy operation involves a few days in hospital. The cone of affected cervical tissue is removed (this can be done surgically or with a laser) and sent for analysis, which takes about a fortnight. Providing it comes back with an all-clear, showing that there has been no spread of abnormal cells (and this will be the case for the vast majority of women), you will now be cured and subject only to the same follow-up as for the other treatments.

Sometimes surgery causes complications. For instance, it may block the opening of the external os and so prevent the flow of menstrual blood, in which case a small operation is done to open it up again. Or it may weaken the muscle of the internal cervical os so that a pregnant woman risks losing her baby after about the twelfth week. If you have had a cone biopsy and later become pregnant, it is important to tell the doctor at your first antenatal visit so that he or she can keep a careful eye on your os. If it shows signs of opening, a temporary stitch can be inserted in your cervix at about the twelfth week to hold the baby in. It is removed shortly before labour is due, and the birth will proceed normally.

Hysterectomy, which means removing the uterus and cervix, is occasionally offered to women who have other gynaecological problems – for instance, troublesome fibroids. Usually these women are older and have completed their families.

REASONS WHY YOU SHOULD GO FOR MORE FREQUENT CERVICAL SCREENING, PREFERABLY EVERY YEAR

You have been on the Pill longer than five years;

You are a heavy smoker;

You or your partner has genital warts;

You have recently changed your sexual partner;

One of you is sleeping with other people at the same time;

You have had an abnormal smear.

WHAT CAUSES AN ABNORMAL SMEAR

As we said at the beginning of this chapter, there are many leads and many suspects, but no positive evidence to link any one of them conclusively with cervical cancer. Smoking; the Pill; several sexual partners; starting sex early; having babies early; a genital infection; a partner's occupation; and sperm have all been suggested; not necessarily as directly causal but certainly as co-factors which could make a woman more vulnerable. Some, like a husband's occupation or sperm, are more speculative than others but what is not in doubt is that a barrier method of contraception – the condom, for instance – provides a more effective protection against infection than the Pill. This becomes very important if you have several sexual partners.

Because of this particular cancer's undoubted link with sex, it has been far too easy to point the finger and suggest that promiscuity is the cause. Someone has suggested that there's only one way we judge promiscuity: you have slept with one more person than I have. Be that as it may, many women who have led exceptionally chaste and faithful lives also develop cervical cancer. Sadly, they may be those who are most at risk because they are the least likely to go for a check-up. They believe that it's 'dirty' to get cervical cancer, a sign that you have lived an immoral life. They may be long past the menopause and believe that nothing can be going on 'down there'. Eighty per cent of the women who develop cervical cancer are over forty and most of them will not have had a smear.

That said, cervical cancer is showing a worrying increase among younger women, so much so that some doctors are talking about an epidemic.

Cherchez l'homme: The HPV wart virus, which we have already mentioned, seems to be significant and this is difficult to deal with, because both men and women may carry it unawares. The warts are often invisible to the naked eye, showing up only under the microscope and then proving quite difficult to treat. If a woman shows signs of HPV virus in her smear, her partner should also be examined. Unfortunately, there is no effective treatment as yet for men with this infection but he can use a condom to prevent reinfecting his partner. This virus can lie dormant for a long time and he may not have been responsible for passing on the infection; it could have been a previous partner.

A husband's occupation also seems to have some bearing. Jean Robinson, a lay member of the General Medical Council and a tireless campaigner on women's health issues, has done interesting research on the relationship between certain male jobs and high rates of cervical cancer in the men's wives.[3]

The relevance of early sexual activity and an early pregnancy may be connected with hormonal changes. Puberty and pregnancy are both periods of great hormonal turmoil and the immature cervix may be subjected to an onslaught it cannot withstand. Another factor which could play a part to a greater or lesser degree − if only in reducing the body's immune defences and thus making it less resistant to infection − is smoking. Women who smoke more than a pack a day are ten times more likely to develop cervical cancer; men who smoke are more likely to have penile warts. Nicotine attacks and weakens certain immune defensive cells in the cervical mucus. (More about this in chapter 15.)

POSITIVE SMEAR, POSITIVE THINKING

It is a shock to be told that you have a positive smear. The immediate fear is cancer, even though very few women with abnormal smears will develop it. A host of fears and suspicions floods your mind. Why have you got this? Does it mean you're going to die? What are people going to say or think, because this comes from sex, doesn't it? Who gave it to you? Can you really get rid of it? . . . and so on.

Women of any age often say they feel defiled and ashamed, as if it were their fault; they are made to feel that they have been promiscuous. The media are frequently blamed for whipping up public feeling by carrying stories laden with prurient suggestions about the causes of pre-cervical cancer. Journalists, unfortunately, all too often take their lead unquestioningly from the doctors who feed them their personal views along with the information. You only have to read the medical literature and hear women's own accounts of their experience as they go through the screening and treatment process to know that health professionals can sometimes be quite condemnatory in their attitudes, or just plain insensitive.

The examination is inelegant and intimate and for most women unavoidably embarrassing, so they need to have their emotional as well as their physical privacy respected. It is inexcusable to have people wandering in and out, or unexplained extras attending to observe what is going on. If it is not done with care and consideration the treatment can make a woman feel, quite apart from physical pain, 'trauma, depression, vulnerability, and violation associated with invasion of "private space" '.[4]

Talking to other women who have been through a similar experience, joining a support group or reading a helpful book like Susan Quilliam's *Positive Smear* are all ways to help you

get through this difficult time. There are also some women's
health groups (see Resources) which will give you good
information and put you in touch with other women who
can help, including a counsellor if that is what you feel you
need.

Don't leave your partner out of all this, or blame him too
quickly. He may be feeling as guilty and anxious as you. This
is a time to talk through your emotions, and particularly how
you feel about your relationship with him. Given that you
value it and wish to keep it going, instead of recriminations
see this as an opportunity to restore and consolidate it.

It may also be a good time to think about certain aspects
of your lifestyle. In this unhappy era of AIDS we are surely
all aware that there is something called safe sex. The condom
is the most effective protective against infection and the
diaphragm (cap) worn by the woman, especially if used with
a spermicide, is the next best. Anyone you sleep with probably
slept with other people before they met you. Even if you have
had only one or two sexual partners, they and your present
partner may have had many more. Unless you have been
settled into a monogamous relationship for many years, there
is always a risk that you may pick up a more or less serious
infection from your partner. Using a barrier method of
contraception is one positive precaution; the other is to make
sure you have smears taken annually.

Many women find that the experience of a positive smear
has a positive effect on their lives. It obliges them to take
stock of what they are doing, and they use the time to
reconsider their priorities and directions. They may decide
that they want to take more responsibility for their health.
Improving your diet, taking more exercise, cutting down on
the smoking (more about that in chapter 15) are all positive
ways to make you feel not only better in yourself but more in
control of your life.

There is good news too for women who have had a positive
smear and successful treatment. There is now very convincing
evidence, based on long-term follow-up studies, to show that

these women are very unlikely to have a recurrence of the problem.

CANCER OF THE CERVIX

Unfortunately, some women are going to develop cervical cancer. There are just a few rare cancers which occur in the cervical area without warning, but the most common form of cervical cancer (between 90 and 95 per cent) is the one affecting the squamous cells, and this is the one which, as we have seen, can be detected at an early pre-cancerous stage by screening.

Often there are no symptoms indicating the presence of cervical cancer. Some women may notice irregular menstrual bleeding or vaginal discharge, but these could be caused by many other less serious conditions. However, you should always report any unusual symptom or pain to your doctor because, like most other cancers, the sooner cervical cancer is detected, the better the chance of cure.

The colposcopy may be sufficient to show that cancer is present, but often a cone biopsy is also done. Once the cancer has been discovered, the next step for the doctor is to establish how far it has spread. There are several tests for this and the treatment will be planned on the basis of the results.

The blood, heart and chest are routinely examined. Kidney and bladder function are checked with an *intravenous urogram* or *pyelogram (IVU or IVP)*; this is done by injecting a dye into the arm. It is X-rayed as it passes through the body; this will show up any abnormal changes in the kidneys or urinary system. A *pelvic scan* will be looking for signs of tumour spread in the whole area and you will possibly also have a *lymphangiogram*, using a dye in rather the same way as for a urogram. This is to check the state of the lymph nodes in the pelvis and abdomen. As in breast cancer, their involvement is an indicator of whether the disease has become metastatic. Finally, the surgeon may decide to do an internal examination under general anaesthetic to verify the precise degree of tumour spread. Occasionally a *pelvic ultrasound* is also done for the same reason. This is a painless procedure which is also used for other uterine examinations (see chapter 13).

Once all or most of these tests have been done – it depends on the suspected spread of the cancer – the doctor is able to 'stage' the cancer and plan the treatment accordingly. There are four stages, progressing in gravity from one to four:

> *Stage 1A.* The cancer has only just penetrated the basement membrane, no more than 5 millimetres. This is called micro-invasive cancer and if it is caught at this stage, the outlook for cure is very good. Somewhere between 80 and 90 per cent of women will survive beyond five years, and the vast majority beyond ten years.

Treatment at this stage can be either a cone biopsy – often used for younger women who have not yet had children, and safe if the spread is very limited. Alternatively, it will be a radical hysterectomy called 'Wertheim' or 'Meig' after the Austrian and American surgeons respectively who pioneered it. This takes longer than the usual hysterectomy because in addition to removing the cervix, uterus and possibly a small part of the top of the vagina it also involves taking out the pelvic lymph nodes, which are close to the bladder and urethra (the tube through which you pass urine). This operation means that a woman will not be able to have any more children, but if she is pre-menopausal and her ovaries are healthy, the doctor will keep them so that she does not have the extra problems of an artificial menopause.

> *Stage 1B.* The cancer has spread, but it is still confined to the uterus.

> *Stage 2A.* The cancer has spread a little way beyond the womb into the vagina.

For both these stages, a hysterectomy as above is possible, or radiotherapy. On the whole doctors prefer to do surgery if they can, particularly on younger women, because radiotherapy can affect the vagina, causing it to shrink. This isn't irremediable; regular intercourse or the use of a vaginal dilator and oestrogen cream will help, but if it can be avoided, so much the better. Radiotherapy also affects the ovaries – you can't avoid an artificial menopause – and it may cause some problems with bowel and bladder function.

Radiotherapy is applied either externally or internally, and sometimes in combination. When it is done internally, a radioactive rod is inserted into the uterus and vagina, where it stays for one to three days. During this time you have to be in a room on your own and nurses and visitors will wear protective clothing because you are slightly radioactive. This wears off as soon as the rod is removed.

Stage 2B. The cancer has spread into tissue around the cervix (parametrium). Radiotherapy is the treatment of choice.

Stage 3. The cancer has spread well beyond the uterus but it is still confined within the pelvis. Again, radiotherapy is the treatment of choice.

Stage 4. The cancer has spread outside the pelvic area into other organs like the bladder and the rectum. Radiotherapy is the treatment of choice, but eventually it may be necessary to do extensive surgery, removing organs like the bladder and rectum.

Chemotherapy is sometimes used for advanced cervical cancer. It may also be given after surgery or radiotherapy as a systemic treatment if the lymph nodes are cancerous.

Radiotherapy can make you feel nauseous, tired and depressed. It can also give you cystitis and diarrhoea, but all this stops once the treatment is over. Occasionally there is some vaginal bleeding even after the treatment, which is part of the healing process, but you should always report it to your doctor. The external treatment is done in much the same way as for breast cancer, with daily visits to the hospital over a few weeks.

The further the cancer has spread, the more difficult it is to cure. Even so, the five-year survival rate for cervical cancer at Stage 2 is approximately 60 per cent, which compares favourably with many other cancers. Rates for later stages are significantly lower, with women who are discovered at Stage 4 having no more than a 10 per cent hope of survival after five years. Most of the women with later stages of cancer are in their fifties and sixties.

These dismal facts emphasise yet again how important it is to have a regular smear. By taking this simple precaution you can avoid this disease. You who are reading this may already be convinced and attend regularly for a smear, but cast around among your older women relatives and friends. If you suspect that they are being squeamish or head-in-the-sand about this test, try to use your powers of persuasion to change their attitude. Your action could save a life.

[13]

The secret enemy

Like any other part of the body, a woman's reproductive and genital organs are vulnerable to cancers of various kinds. Since these organs are mostly internal, the disease can establish itself and spread before there are any visible symptoms. Most of these cancers appear in post-menopausal, often quite elderly women and the first indication they may have of something wrong is unexpected and copious vaginal bleeding, a smelly discharge or pain in the pelvic or abdominal area. Although these cancers cannot be screened – with the exception of ovarian cancer, and that is still in the experimental stage – it is important to report anything unusual to your doctor as soon as possible, even if you are feeling quite well in yourself. Typically of all cancers, these too develop in stages and the earlier they are detected and treated, the higher your chances of cure. One way a doctor can check the condition of your uterus and ovaries is by doing a bimanual pelvic examination: he feels your uterus and ovaries through both vagina and rectum. This is usually done only by a gynaecologist.

ENDOMETRIAL (UTERINE) CANCER

The endometrium is the inner lining of the uterus, some of which is shed every month during a woman's fertile years if she has not become pregnant. After the menopause, when the ovaries stop producing oestrogen and progesterone, this shedding (menstruation) also ceases because the uterus is no longer preparing itself for pregnancy. The endometrium, however, remains susceptible to oestrogen stimulation; this occurs naturally and in some women more than others; it can be heightened still more if a woman is on hormone replacement therapy.

Endometrial cancer is a common gynaecological cancer – it comprises 13 per cent of all female cancers – and it is hormone-dependent. Oestrogen is the catalysing agent and post-menopausal women between fifty-five and seventy are most at risk. Other risk factors include being overweight, never having children, having a late menopause (after fifty-two), and a family history of endometrial or breast cancer. How can oestrogen have this effect if the ovaries are no longer producing it?

In several ways. The adrenal glands produce some oestrogen in adipose tissue; the more obese the woman, the higher the level of circulating oestrogen but at the same time, because she is no longer ovulating, there is no counteractive progesterone to mitigate the effects of this endogenous oestrogen. The small number of pre-menopausal women who develop endometrial cancer (about 20 per cent of the annual 3,700, and only 3 per cent of those will be under forty) tend to have some condition causing them not to ovulate or to produce exceptional amounts of oestrogen.

Women who take hormone replacement therapy to counteract the effects of menopause will continue to have a light monthly bleed. In America, where HRT has been available since the early sixties, there was for a while a sharp increase in endometrial cancer until it was realised that this was due to high doses of 'unopposed' exogenous oestrogen – that is to say, it was not being counterbalanced by progestogen. British doctors, who generally prefer to err on the side of caution, have been slow to prescribe HRT and have accordingly been castigated by many women for their conservatism, but at least the annual incidence of endometrial cancer has remained steady in this country. Today, thanks to research and several trials, HRT is much better understood and its risks and benefits have already been discussed in chapter 2. There are advantages in taking the present much more carefully monitored dosages, particularly if you are suffering from uncomfortable menopausal symptoms, but women with a family history of endometrial cancer should not consider it.

Post-menopausal bleeding is the most usual symptom of endometrial cancer and it should always be reported immediately. In pre-menopausal women it is more likely to present as bleeding between normal periods. Occasionally, there is also a watery discharge. As this is a cancer with a very high five-year survival rate – somewhere between 70 and 95 per cent if it is discovered early enough – it is most important not to delay your visit to your doctor.

The treatment for endometrial cancer depends very much on the stage and the type of tumour and needs to be highly individualised for each patient. An abnormal smear sometimes indicates cancerous endometrial cells but is not a very reliable indicator, and it will be necessary for the doctor to do a biopsy as well. This will take the form of a D and C (dilatation and curettage of the uterus under general anaesthetic). The age and general health of the woman are important factors; many women with this cancer have to contend with other serious medical problems like high blood pressure and diabetes.

Surgery is the treatment of choice, and for some early cancers it may be all that is necessary – a hysterectomy which includes removing the fallopian tubes and ovaries.

Radiotherapy is seldom used at this stage but if the cancer is more advanced it can be administered either externally by beam or internally with radium rods, somewhat as described for cervical cancer. In some cases, radiotherapy may be used on its own.

Hormone (progesterone) therapy has been used as an adjuvant treatment for early endometrial cancer instead of radiotherapy, but this is regarded as controversial and it is more usually given for advanced cancer or when it recurs. The progesterone has to be taken for at least twelve weeks before the doctor can tell whether it is succeeding in shrinking the tumour; if it is, it will have to be continued indefinitely. An alternative is tamoxifen, which is now considered to be equally good and is often given to patients who either do not respond to progesterone or have relapsed.

Chemotherapy is regarded as experimental and of doubtful benefit for this particular cancer; it is, therefore, seldom used.

The treatment options for this cancer are fairly straight-forward, particularly if it is detected at an early stage but, as we said earlier, other factors about the woman's general state of health will also have to be taken into account when the doctor discusses her treatment plan with her.

OVARIAN CANCER

Unfortunately, this is a cancer with a higher incidence – something over 5,000 new cases diagnosed every year – and a higher mortality rate than for cervical and endometrial cancer combined. It is the fifth most common female cancer and every year in Britain more than 4,000 women die from it, most of them because their disease is already at an advanced stage by the time they have consulted a doctor.

The tragedy is that in the main they would have had no reason to come earlier: the symptoms of ovarian cancer are vague and easily attributed to indigestion or gaining a bit of middle-aged spread. Pain is very seldom a feature. There may be a sense of bloatedness, sometimes nausea, bouts of consti-pation or diarrhoea, or a need to pass water more often. Even the normally detached scientists who write medical textbooks allow themselves uncharacteristic emotions here, using such phrases as 'the silent killer', 'this sinister malignancy' or 'the enigma' to describe its secret growth. On the whole it is an early post-menopausal cancer, though women in their twen-ties and thirties can also get it and these younger women tend to have a better prognosis, possibly because it appears easier to pick up the disease at an early stage in this age group.

It is difficult to identify a high-risk group although there does seem to be a slight familial link, this being a cancer known to occur in succeeding generations. Women who do not have children are definitely more at risk. Conversely, there is a clear benefit from being on the Pill – the longer the better – and this benefit extends to endometrial cancer as well.[1,2] Where precisely this leaves women is not so clear. Heads, you want neither ovarian nor endometrial cancer and maybe the Pill will protect you. Tails, no more do you want breast or cervical cancer but here, as we have already seen in earlier chapters, the evidence about the Pill's effects is much more equivocal and cannot be said to be pointing in a favourable direction. Better-off women living in the Western industrialised countries are more vulnerable than Eastern women. However, just as for breast cancer, Japanese women provide an interesting exception. Those who move to North America soon lose their apparent immunity to ovarian cancer and by the third generation they are as susceptible as their Western sisters, suggesting once again an environmental factor.

Finding a good screening test is what everyone is now pinning their hopes on. There are several trials currently in progress in this country. First in the field was the team at King's College Hospital, London, who, in the early eighties, screened 5,479 self-selected women over the age of forty-five annually for three years with ultrasound. This is a painless procedure which takes about twenty minutes. You drink at least two pints of fluid beforehand to fill your bladder; thus inflated, it pushes the ovaries into view. Your stomach is rubbed with a cream and then a flat probe is run gently all over it, 'sounding' it rather like a ship sounds the depths and throwing a picture of your internal organs up on the screen.

The preliminary results of this trial show that following the ultrasound a total of 379 women were given further exploratory examinations, either by laparascopy or laparotomy, to discover the state of their ovaries.[3] Of these, five had cancer, twelve had 'pre-malignant symptoms' and four had metastatic cancer. The rest would have had cysts and other benign lesions or possibly temporarily enlarged ovaries reflecting hormonal changes that would have reverted to normal in due course. Against the five lives definitely saved has to be weighed the cost of investigating a few hundred women under general anaesthetic and the distress caused to four women told they had advanced cancer possibly a few months, even a year or more, before it would otherwise have been discovered.

A different screening method, being tried out at the London Hospital, consists of a blood test, a questionnaire and a pelvic examination. If the blood test establishes the presence of a protein called CA 125, which is produced by tumour cells and is in the blood of 90 per cent of women ultimately diagnosed with ovarian cancer, the woman is asked back to have an ultrasound. The researchers make the point that no individual screening test is 100 per cent specific but the combination of these three tests, with ultrasound being brought in as a back-up procedure, 'offers the most hope of a specific and sensitive method for early detection'.[4]

This trial is running now and needs to recruit at least 30,000 women if it is to produce valid results. The test costs something under £5 per woman and is being privately funded because the NHS doesn't see ovarian screening as a priority. Yet if this simple test does work, it could be offered to women at the same time as they go for their breast screen. Indeed, it's hard to see why this could not be done now, had we more flexible policy-makers and possibly also doctors who were more prepared to co-operate with their colleagues. Meanwhile, if you are eligible – over forty-five and have not had a period for at least a year – and would like to participate, contact the Ovary Screening Clinic, the London Hospital, Whitechapel E1 1BB (telephone 01-377 7674).

Both the Cancer Research Campaign and the Imperial Cancer Research Fund are also funding trials for ovarian cancer screening, so there is some hope that there will be a positive advance in the next decade.

Treatment for this cancer must be individually planned because there are so many different kinds of ovarian tumour and much depends on the degree of spread. As for the other cancers of the reproductive organs several preliminary tests are necessary: an *abdominal scan,* an *intravenous urogram* and a *lymphangiogram,* as described in chapter 12. If fluid has collected in the abdomen – this is called ascites and is a common phenomenon of ovarian cancer – a sample will be drawn off with a fine needle into a syringe to test for cancer cells. This is called *abdominal fluid aspiration.* You will also have to have a *barium enema* to enable your bowel to be X-rayed. This is quite a lengthy procedure, involving some preparation before you arrive at the hospital: eating a simple diet and taking a laxative to empty your bowels, for instance. In the X-ray department the nurse will wash out your colon with warm water and then give you an enema consisting of barium and air. X-rays are taken of the barium as it passes through your bowel, and these will show up any abnormalities.

If the cancer has been found really early, a hysterectomy, including removing your fallopian tubes and ovaries, may be all that is necessary. That may sound like a lot too much and none of it good but survival rates for ovarian cancer removed at this stage are over 90 per cent. Given that the prognosis for later stage ovarian cancer is all too often a poor one, surgery will seem a price worth paying, especially if your childbearing days are over. Sometimes, when the patient is a younger pre-menopausal woman who would still like children, the doctor will try to save one ovary and one fallopian tube, if they are in a healthy condition, so that she retains a chance of conceiving. Since she has a higher-than-average risk of developing cancer in the remaining ovary at a later stage, most doctors will recommend that it be removed after she has completed childbearing.

Having a hysterectomy should not affect your sex life,

although it will make you feel tired and possibly uninterested in sex for a while. Women vary enormously in their emotional reaction to this operation. Some feel relieved and happy: the fear of pregnancy has been removed from them; others, even older women who are past the menopause, may feel a sense of bereavement at losing part of their womanly equipment. (See further reading for some helpful books.) Physically, you should convalesce for a few weeks after the operation, resuming your normal life slowly and not undertaking too many heavy physical tasks. Most women find they are able to resume intercourse about six weeks after the operation, and if there are problems with a dry vagina caused by the sudden cessation of oestrogen, a lubricant like KY jelly or a vaginal oestrogen cream will help.

Surgery is almost always the treatment of choice for ovarian cancer, the aim being to reduce the tumour mass – which may be very large – as much as possible. Although small spots of disease will remain throughout the abdomen, this process of 'debulking' the tumour is now known to be very important, no matter how advanced the cancer, because it greatly improves the patient's subsequent response to chemotherapy.

Chemotherapy is given either orally or intravenously (injection into a vein). For ovarian cancer it is usually a single drug – Cisplatinum or its analogue Carboplatin. This latter drug has far less severe side-effects than Cisplatinum, causing little nausea and no damage to the kidneys or numbness in the hands or feet. Neither drug causes hair loss. Many patients can be treated quite successfully with tablets which they take daily for a few weeks and then stop for a few weeks, over a period of several months.

Radiotherapy has a limited role in the treatment of this cancer. It has to be used with some caution because it can permanently damage neighbouring organs in the abdominal cavity like the liver, the bowels and the bladder, all of which are more sensitive to radiotherapy than to the disease itself. British doctors in particular use radiotherapy much more carefully than they used to and they are very aware of these risks, so you should feel reassured if you are offered it as part of your total treatment. No one has yet hit on the optimum combination of adjuvant treatments for ovarian cancer, but chemotherapy is undoubtedly producing better results for woman with advanced disease.

Although the picture by and large is still a gloomy one for ovarian cancer – the five-year survival rate is only 28 per cent – there are glimmers of hope. The treatments are improving and many more women who would once have been regarded as inoperable are responding well to treatments and living longer, with a reasonable quality of life. It is in screening, however – and specifically in finding a reliable, not too onerous test – that our best hope lies, because this cancer has a good prognosis if it is found really early.

RARE CANCERS OF THE REPRODUCTIVE AND SEXUAL ORGANS

These include the vulva, vagina and fallopian tubes. Cancer of the vulva usually occurs in quite elderly women, but recently it has been appearing more often in younger women. It is a slow-growing cancer and is often preceded by a period when the vulva feels very itchy and there may be a sore patch on the labia (lips of the vulva). Providing it is caught at an early stage, the five-year survival rate is good and surgery is usually the only treatment necessary, but sometimes it will be followed up by radiotherapy.

The operation for cancer of the vulva is called a vulvectomy and it involves removing all the affected area, probably including the clitoris and possibly also lymph glands in the groin. Some skin grafting may be necessary and for ten days after the operation the woman will have to have a catheter in her urethra to drain urine from the bladder.

Clearly for any woman with an active sexual life, this is an operation with serious psychological implications. Her sense of her own sexuality is entwined with her perception of her body image, and now it has been irrevocably altered. The labia will have been removed, making her vulva look flat and therefore different. Sometimes the vaginal entrance is tighter and the vagina itself a bit shorter. Orgasm will obviously no longer be possible through the clitoris if it has been removed, but women who were orgasmic before their operation can often continue to experience orgasm, even though the sensation comes from inside rather than outside the vagina.

Understandably, many women find it hard to come to terms with their changed image and may fear the reactions of their sexual partner. This is a time when a woman can benefit very much from counselling, and an American study has shown that counselled women are able to renew their sexual and everyday life much more rapidly than women denied this help.[5] Sometimes it is enough to talk through your worries and fears with an ordinarily trained counsellor, but it may be better for some women to consult a sex therapist. (See Resources for addresses or write to CancerLink for their booklet *Body Image, Sexuality and Cancer*.)

Vaginal cancer is even rarer but came dramatically into prominence in the seventies, particularly in the United States, with the revelation that some daughters of women who had taken Diethylstilboestrol (DES), a synthetic oestrogen, during their pregnancy to avoid a miscarriage were developing a form of vaginal cancer in their teens and early twenties. Further investigation has shown that many of these women also have uterine abnormalities which make childbearing more difficult. Many have undergone radical surgery and the suffering, psychological as well as physical, both they and their mothers continue to endure is severe.

Again the innate conservatism of British doctors has served to protect their patients because they were never very enthusiastic about using DES for treating miscarriages and stopped altogether in the mid 1950s, whereas the Americans continued using it until well into the 1970s. Since vaginal cancer mostly affects young women in their teens and early twenties, those in Britain who could have been in danger of being affected are now likely to have passed the 'at risk' age.

The story of DES, which has been used in many other ways – for fattening chickens, in HRT and to stop lactation, to give but a few examples – has not yet ended. Its connection with the rising rate of breast cancer is under investigation, particularly in the mothers who took DES. It may also be causative in the increase of other female genital cancers. Another neglected area of enquiry which is now being investigated is the effects it may have had on the sons of these same women. All in all – as a fascinating book called *To Do No Harm*, by two American psychiatrists, reveals – this is a modern morality tale about medical myths and miracles from which we could gain much wisdom, even though it is after the event; but no doubt, as usual, we will probably learn little or nothing until the whole disaster repeats itself with another 'wonder drug' or 'medical breakthrough'.

[14]

Black spot

Just one of the many disastrous effects of the gaping hole torn in the ozone layer is that we are losing our protection from ultraviolet radiation: those powerful rays which cause sunburn, increasingly with lethal consequences. There is evidence to suggest that even one bad exposure in childhood or teens could be a significant risk factor for developing malignant melanoma years later.

Once a rare form of skin cancer, malignant melanoma is now increasing by around 5 per cent a year. In Britain, 1,733 women developed it in 1984 (latest available figures), which is more than double the number of men, though for some as yet unexplained reason younger women have a better prognosis than men. There is a suggestion that it may be hormone-related, because after the menopause the male–female ratio evens up, but this is not a cancer to take lightly at any age. Is it ever? Malignant melanoma must be reported really early if it is to be cured. Then – but then only – the survival rate is excellent: 92 per cent will be well, with no signs of recurrence, after five years.

'Devastating, aggressive, deadly' is the way it has been described by Sidney Hurwitz, an American dermatologist. He would like to see women's magazines and other fashion arbiters lead a return to the delicate porcelain complexions of our Edwardian grandmothers, ladies who were shaded by their parasols and would have died rather than expose a square inch of skin to the sun. We blonde blue-eyed Northerners who yearn to turn our sun-starved flesh from lobster pink to golden brown on an annual fortnight's holiday in the Southern sun are the ones most at risk – even more so if we are of Celtic origin, with the characteristic reddish hair and thin freckled skin which always tans badly. Read on and you may wonder why anyone bothers to try.

There are four types of malignant melanoma:

Superficial spreading, which is the most common, looks like a brown irregularly shaped patch, at least one centimetre across and often larger, mostly on the leg in women and on the trunk in men. It grows slowly to begin with but later, if you look closely at it, you will see it has variously coloured pigmentation – brown, black, blue, red and white – and a slightly raised surface.

Nodular, the next most common variety, usually appears on the trunk as a fast-growing raised black or reddish nodule. It will have a ragged edge and be irregularly pigmented – colours include blue-black, blue-grey and reddish blue. If left it will ulcerate, and it is highly dangerous because it grows vertically into the body – taking root, as it were.

Lentigo maligna appears most often as a large, flat brown mark on the cheeks of old people, but also on other parts of the face and body which have been habitually exposed to the sun. It spreads slowly in its early phase but becomes invasively malignant when it thickens into a nodule which turns black or blue and white. It will start to crust and eventually ulcerate if left.

Acral lentiginous, is the rarest type in Britain, appears as a spreading brown patch on the sole of the foot, the palm of the hand, or under a nail.

Warning signs which you must report immediately to your doctor include:

any change at all in the shape or colour of a mole;

any new mole or patch on the body anywhere, especially one which seems to be growing rapidly;

an itching or 'creeping' sensation round the edges of a mole (an early sign of malignancy);

bleeding, oozing or crusting (all earlyish signs);

ulceration and new moles growing round the original one (later signs);

a hairy mole which loses its hair.

Naturally dark-skinned people are far less likely to contract malignant melanoma because the extra melanin in their skin affords them good protection. Nature isn't stupid, since they also mostly live in the hottest parts of the world. Other people who are at high risk, in addition to those already mentioned, include:

anyone who has a lot of normal moles on their body (over fifty);

anyone who has many unusual-looking moles;

anyone with a family history of melanoma;

anyone who has already had one malignant melanoma.

Until recently GPs have not been very good at recognising early malignant melanoma, partly because individually they would not have seen many cases during the course of their practice. But now there is a national campaign, funded by the Cancer Research Campaign, to increase their awareness as well as that of the general public.[1] It is far better that you be referred to a consultant for something which turns out to be harmless than that you wait a year because it seems 'silly to make a fuss about something so small' or because your doctor has failed to recognise any of the warning signs.

DIAGNOSIS AND TREATMENT

If your GP suspects something could be wrong, you will be sent immediately to a specialist clinic. If you are unhappy about a mole but your GP doesn't seem too perturbed, insist on a second opinion. Time is of the essence with this cancer, particularly once you have noticed any changes.

At the clinic, the mole will be removed and sent to the laboratory for measurement and histological analysis. It is measured according to the Breslow scale to see how thick it is; if it is less than one millimetre it has a very good prognosis – over 90 per cent cure after five years for both men and women. However thin the melanoma is, you may still have to go into hospital because the doctor will want to remove surrounding normal tissue of at least the diameter of a 10 pence piece, and this will mean a small skin graft. Nowadays, the surgery is considerably less traumatic and scarring than it used to be even a few years ago because so much less tissue is removed. Many surgeons operate on the principle of one centimetre of normal skin around the tumour for each millimetre it has penetrated, with a maximum margin of three centimetres.

If the tumour is somewhere between 1.5 and 3.5 milli-metres thick, lymph nodes may also be removed as a precaution against further spread, but this is regarded as a controversial treatment in Britain. Doctors here are awaiting the results of clinical trials. Meanwhile lymphoedema is a hazard with this procedure, especially when the melanoma is on an arm or leg. On the other hand, melanoma on a limb carries a better overall prognosis.

Neither chemotherapy nor radiotherapy works very well on this particular cancer, although the latter is used to palliate advanced disease.

Follow-up is very important. At first you will visit the clinic every three months and then, after two years or so, every six months. This will probably continue for at least ten years.

Clearly, between visits it is important to do your own self-examination and report anything untoward at once.

'I could never actually believe that something on my foot could kill me,' says a woman who spent about six months 'being aware' of a mole on her ankle before she went to her GP, who was sceptical that anything was wrong. 'He said I'd better see a specialist if I was worried but I was only scared when they talked about an emergency.' She was taken straight into hospital and was fortunate enough to have an early contained melanoma.

It is not only important to protect yourself against over-exposure to the sun; your children are equally vulnerable. What was once regarded as old-fashioned advice from our grandmothers to wear vests and sunhats at all times is now proving to be wise and sensible after all. Moderate, steady exposure is much better than intensive bouts of sunbathing under a burning sky. Any sporting activity where the skin is exposed to high levels of ultraviolet radiation, whether on the mountains, by the sea or in the country, carries an increased risk. We should all use sunscreens and avoid artificial tanning creams which, despite their claims, are not 'safer than the sun'.

PART THREE

Your life in your hands

[15]

The last puff

THE SMOKING CONNECTION

It takes the average smoker approximately five minutes to go through the routine of lighting up, pulling the deep drag, or puffing frantically – depending on your style – and then smoking down to the butt. Those five 'satisfying' minutes could be more costly than you might imagine. It's not just a matter of burning a hole in your purse: it has been estimated that each cigarette burns five non-returnable minutes off your life . . . quite literally. If you do your sums you will find that twenty cigarettes a day means that twenty-five days of your life are going up in smoke *every* year! Many more, of course, if you are a two- or three-pack-daily smoker – that could mean dying prematurely by ten to fifteen years.

A cigarette smoker runs a one in four risk of dying from her habit. Heart disease and lung cancer are the chief killers. From being a rare, hardly ever seen cancer at the beginning of this century, lung cancer is now the cause of more than 40,000 deaths a year (men and women) and it has become the second most common cancer in women. The annual death rate for women (11,881 in 1987) has risen by 27 per cent since 1979. That is almost three times the rate of breast cancer in the same period, and medical statisticians are predicting that by the year 2000 lung cancer will have overtaken breast cancer as the major cause of female deaths from cancer. It has already happened in Scotland. Lung cancer has a long latent period and this recent dramatic rise in women's death dates from the forties, fifties and sixties when women started smoking in earnest.

Other cancers are also smoking-related. Cancers of the tongue, jaw, throat and oesophagus are all implicated, as are organs much further away like the bladder, pancreas and cervix. This is because tobacco smoke contains carcinogenic substances which are absorbed from the lungs into the bloodstream and carried round the body. Why smokers should be more likely to have positive smears and indications of CIN III has long been a puzzle – at least until recently, when an important paper in *The Lancet* finally threw up some good evidence suggesting one possibility: a decreased immunity.[1]

To put it very basically, it has been discovered that smokers have fewer Langerhans' cells in their cervical cell lining, probably because nicotine or some other chemical by-product of smoking has infiltrated the cervical mucus and killed them off. Langerhans' cells are the ones which provide immune protection: for instance, from viral infections like HPV 16. Although this particular connection has not yet been conclusively proved, it does now seem probable that smoking is the potent co-factor with human papilloma virus which causes some forms of cervical dysplasia. This could also explain why there are also women with the virus who do not go on to develop CIN. Is it because they do not smoke?

We shall have to await the results of further studies before we can be certain that this is so. Meanwhile, even if we do not yet completely understand the process which causes the change, it should be enough to know that there is a sinister connection between CIG and CIN: smoking twenty cigarettes a day increases your risk of CIN seven times; forty cigarettes a day puts it up to fourteen times.

OTHER UNDESIRABLE SIDE-EFFECTS

Although this book is about cancer, smoking damages our health in so many other ways that a brief consideration of these risks may help those of us who are still struggling to give up the weed. Heart disease, strokes, chronic bronchitis and emphysema – a very disabling lung disease which leaves the victim painfully short of breath – can all be caused by smoking. And even if it doesn't quite kill you, there are a number of ways smoking can make your life a misery, particularly if you are a woman.

Studies have shown that smoking is directly toxic to the ovaries, frequently causing cysts and upsetting the hormonal cycle. Women smokers are more likely to be infertile, have an early menopause, and develop osteoporosis (brittle bones) after the menopause. Smoking can also make you look old and hairy before your time, because smokers tend to get more wrinkles – the skin loses its elasticity earlier – and grow excessive facial hair.

This catalogue of woe does not end with the harm you can do yourself. Every time a pregnant woman inhales a cigarette she is effectively starving her baby because the nicotine closes down the blood vessels through which the foetus receives its nourishment from the mother. At best she risks having an underweight, frail baby, or she may give birth prematurely; at worst, she may even lose her baby in its early weeks. It is also thought that heavy smokers may be increasing the risk of their child developing leukaemia later on.

Children who are brought up by smoking parents are much more susceptible to colds and chest infections. It has been estimated that a child living in a smoke-filled home is itself 'smoking' the equivalent of 150 cigarettes a year. Passive smoking, as this is called, is reckoned to cause about 200 deaths a year in the adult population.

SO WHY DO WE DO IT?

Rationality has nothing to do with it, and feeling guilty just makes some people smoke more. Human beings have always been inventive about finding excuses to justify doing something which is bad for them. Knowing that something is dangerous, even that it's capable of killing, is not the same as believing it will actually happen to you.

Physical addiction is only part of the reason. It takes a mere three or four days for nicotine, which is the addictive substance in a cigarette, to clear out of the system and, as most ex-smokers will confirm, with every day that goes by, the acute physical craving diminishes. This is not to deny that some people will suffer quite severe withdrawal symptoms for weeks or even months after they have stopped smoking. Stomach upsets, constipation, dizziness, headaches, nausea, lack of concentration are all common physical reactions while the toxins drain out of the body. Unpleasant though these are, they do eventually disappear and you have only to hear an established ex-smoker waxing lyrical about how much better he or she feels to realise that the long-term physical benefits far outweigh any initial discomforts.

The real addiction is psychological, and that is much more difficult to root out. There are many different types of smokers, but what they share in common is a personal conviction that smoking is in some way necessary to them. If you started smoking as a teenager (and most habitual smokers did) you probably began out of curiosity or to keep up with your friends, and then continued because you felt it made you look grown-up and sophisticated. It is surprising how significant that first cigarette can be – many people remember the occasion as vividly as losing their virginity.

Adult smokers often continue smoking to give themselves social confidence. They walk into a crowded room full of strangers or into some situation which makes them feel uncomfortable, so they light up a cigarette and immediately they feel at ease.

Research has shown that there are some quite important differences between the sexes.[2] Men, it seems, are more likely to smoke because they think it enhances their image or they take a sensuous pleasure in the whole ritual, particularly the oral contact. (There's an attractive – though unproven – theory that breastfed babies are less likely to become smokers because they were able to enjoy full oral satisfaction at the right age.) Men also often use cigarettes as a stimulus to action or as a way of relieving tedium or the monotony of a boring job: 'Smoking helps me to concentrate', or 'get on with the job.'

Women, by contrast, tend to use smoking as a sedative and a stress-reliever. 'It calms my nerves,' 'It helps me relax,' 'I feel I can cope better with a cigarette,' are as likely to be said by the harassed mother who is short of money and on her own all day with young children as by the ambitious female executive who is competing in a man's world and possibly running a family as well as a career. Often women smoke quite deliberately to control emotions which they think are unacceptable – anger, frustration, a sense of helplessness, a feeling that they have no control over their fate.

Divorced, widowed and separated women are more likely to smoke than married women. Women who are unemployed or housebound are also slightly more likely to smoke than women with jobs. According to an analysis of figures put out by the ASH Women and Smoking Group, the type of work a woman does has little bearing on whether or not she smokes, but her husband's occupation does matter. Apparently only 15 per cent of women with professional husbands smoke, whereas 46 per cent of women whose husbands do unskilled manual work will be smokers.[3]

Nurses are an interesting exception. They are well known to have a higher rate of smoking than any other group of working women, yet the evidence is that they know the harmful consequences quite as well as doctors, and believe just as strongly as doctors that they should advise their patients against it. So why do they do it?

Bobbie Jacobson advances a convincing – if depressing – explanation in her book *Beating the Ladykillers*. The hospital set-up, she suggests, is a 'microcosm of male dominance'. Nurses do demanding and highly stressful work, and bear a lot of responsibility at a much younger age than most doctors. Yet the work carries little status, either financially or socially, and when it comes to the important decisions it is invariably the doctor, usually male, who makes them. As nurses know to their cost, they may be praised as angels but they are treated like skivvies, so they are tempted to take out their frustration and anger in smoking. It may not be a sensible reaction, but it is understandable.

A myth which really deserves nailing is the one perpetuated in the Virginia Slim slogan, 'You've come a long way, baby', suggesting that emancipation is complete only when you've got a cigarette dangling from your fingers. This is only the last in a long line of advertising messages which have, over the past half-century, suggested to women that their sex appeal and their competence are enhanced by smoking.

'Keep smoking and keep slim' is another seductive myth which has been promoted over the years. Since model proportions are so admired in our society, this belief makes it very hard for fashion-conscious women to contemplate stopping. It's true that smoking is an appetite-suppressant, and on the whole women smokers are thinner than non-smokers, but only by a couple of pounds! Even if giving up means you do put on half a stone, that extra weight – which need only be temporary – is certainly not going to endanger your health. Unlike the daily pack.

For a minority, weight gain may genuinely be a question of altered metabolism. If this is your problem, a good way of countering it is by going in for some vigorous exercise – easier when you feel fitter. However, the usual reason for women getting fatter when they stop smoking is that, quite unconsciously, they are putting something else into their mouth to replace the cigarette. This is a physical reaction to a psychological need and it indicates that they haven't yet succeeded in overcoming a strong sense of deprivation every time they crave a cigarette.

WATCH YOUR WEIGHT

Each time you find yourself longing for a cigarette, consciously play a trick on yourself:

Drink a glass of water or fruit juice (unsweetened);

Find something else to do with your hands;

Get up and move around;

Do a task which takes both hands – like clearing out your desk or polishing a piece of furniture;

Take a bath;

Think of any other displacement activity which distracts you from the urge to put something into your mouth.

WARNING: It is unwise to substitute carrots or celery sticks or some other low-calorie alternative because you are really treating them like cigarettes. Sooner or later the deception will pall and you will return to your favourite dummy.

STOP THE STARTING

The good news is that the overall number of women smoking has declined from 41 per cent in 1972 to 32 per cent in 1984 (one-fifth) but this is still a lower rate than for men, for whom the decline has been one-third in the same period. The bad news is that a new generation is lighting up. For the first time ever there are more teenage girl smokers (between sixteen and nineteen years old) than boys. About 25 per cent of them are regular smokers, which means they are smoking at least six cigarettes a week; they say they do it mainly for fun and because it makes them feel sophisticated. Girls also frequently mention weight control.

Example obviously matters. Young children of smoking parents will be especially encouraged to think that it is a normal activity, and this puts parents in a weak position when they want to forbid them from experimenting with cigarettes. All the same, if you are a smoking mother don't let that stop you being tough with your daughter if you catch her smoking. You can explain that it's just because you know how bad it is for you that you don't want her to get hooked in the same way. Most children now know that smoking causes cancer, but personal death is so remote in a child's imagination that it is not a fact with which they can readily associate, so try to think of other reasons which will impress them more: the smell, looking silly with a chimney sticking out of your mouth, the waste of money, and so on.

It is not easy, even when you are a non-smoker yourself, to counteract the other powerful influences which will impinge more and more on your children as they grow up. A best friend or a gang of kids who are all smoking will persuade your child that it is wimpish not to join in. A favourite pop star gyrating in clouds of smoke is much more alluring than teacher giving a boring homily in class about the evils of smoking. A sporting idol wearing a T-shirt emblazoned with the name of a particular brand of cigarettes, or an exciting football match which takes place on a pitch surrounded by posters proclaiming a tobacco company's sponsorship, are all insidious ways of getting across the wrong message.

This is not speculation, it is fact based on extensive research into children's habits, attitudes and beliefs about smoking which has been done mainly by Dr Anne Charlton, a director of the Cancer Research Campaign's Education and Child Studies Group. She has now developed an educational programme to meet the three critical stages she has observed in children's smoking history.[4]

Between nine and eleven they tend to go in for experimentation, and this is the stage where parental involvement can be particularly effective, so the children are given an information pack to take home which backs up what they have been learning at school. This is basically an entertainingly written story which explains, in vivid but not frightening detail, the effects of smoking on the human system. When she came to evaluate its success, Dr Charlton was surprised to find that it seemed to work much better with boys and their fathers, many of whom gave up smoking as a result. She is now racking her brains to think up new ways to get through to the mothers, whose smoking habits did not change at all.

At twelve there is a danger that children will be pressured into becoming regular smokers, so for this age group she reinforces the biological information with an excellent teaching pack about the aims and techniques of advertising. It includes inviting the children to create their own advertising campaign which will be attractive enough 'to sell something about as useless as a bundle of dried-up leaves to people so that they can set fire to it in their mouths, for which plenty of other people get paid a lot of money'.

Finally, she has a Stop Smoking programme for sixth formers and college students, who by this stage may already be addicted. It could be used equally well by older, hardened smokers, since it is based on the vital principle 'Know thyself'. Before they do anything else she asks them to keep a smoking diary for a week and answer a questionnaire which helps them to discover which kind of smoker they are: for instance, are they smoking primarily for comfort, or sensation, or pleasure? Is it to reward themselves or give themselves a confidence-booster? There are many other types of smoker and one isn't worse than another, or more of a hopeless case, but if you can at least try to analyse your motives for smoking you have a better chance of hitting on the method which will work for you.

STARTING TO STOP

Give yourself the good news first: you improve your health from the day you stop. Heart risks diminish after only a few weeks. After five years you are almost down to the risk level of non-smokers, and by ten to fifteen years your chances of getting lung cancer are no greater than those of a lifelong non-smoker – in other words, they are minimal.

Draw up a Benefit list for yourself, writing down all the things you know will make you feel better if you give up. Pin it up on your mirror or over your desk: somewhere you will be sure to see it every day, so that you cannot forget about it.

Think about your habits and your daily routine and the

times you always associate with a cigarette. See how you can alter them.

If you've got this far, you've come a long way. Now you are ready to take the big step, which is deciding that you really do want to stop. This is something you have to do for yourself. Other people nagging you, or even you feeling that you ought to stop for the sake of others – perhaps because you feel you should be giving your children a good example – will not be strong enough reasons to carry you through the bad times. *You, and you alone, are your reason for stopping.*

WHICH METHOD?

It's fun hearing about other people's successes, but what works for them may not work for you. Acupuncture, hynotherapy, diet, psychotherapy, chewing gum, or taking a holiday are all possibilities, but don't fall into the trap of thinking that it will happen for you without any real effort. The most important requirement for stopping is that you have decided you want to give up. Don't be discouraged if you falter and fail more than once. If you really want to stop, you will do it eventually.

The cheapest and often quickest way is to do it on your own. That is what most ex-smokers have done, like one woman who, after thirty-five years of smoking forty a day, quietly decided to stop and told no one. She said: 'I suddenly realised that I didn't want to commit suicide.' She keeps a pack of cigarettes in her dressing-table and every now and then she allows herself to slaver longingly over it, but it is six months since she stopped and she feels she is over the hump.

Others find it easier to go on a programme where they can work in a group. There are plenty of books offering help, and ASH (see Resources) can put you in touch with a local support group. It may be ill-health or self-disgust or just a longing to take charge of yourself which makes you seek to kick the habit. Perhaps you are like this woman, who said she was finally tired of being 'so eternally vulnerable. I knew

I had reached the peak of neurotic deprivation when I twice rang a taxi firm at two in the morning to get me a packet of cigarettes.' Or it may be that you find smoking an unaccept-able contradiction in your life. Here you are deeply concerned about the environment, pollution and toxins in your daily diet, yet you are absorbing the worst poison of all – and it is self-inflicted. 'Smoking', said a woman who felt precisely like this, 'numbs the feelings in your heart and chest and anaesthe-tises your emotions. Giving up gives you a chance to feel again.'

Could there be a better promise to offer anyone? Whether you do it on your own, in a support group – which many women find especially helpful – or use one of the complemen-tary methods, hold on to your own particular hope. The triumph of banishing the weed from your life will make you feel ready to tackle anything.

If you don't think you can stop now but you do want to reduce your risk, try . . .

Delaying your first cigarette of the day. For example, when you've brought it forward from first thing in the morning to after breakfast, take it forward again to the mid-morning break, and so on.

Smoking a milder brand. The reduced tar content does mean a little less gunge lining your lungs, but don't fool yourself! It doesn't diminish cardiovascular and other risks.

Buying filter-tipped cigarettes; or use a holder with a built-in filter, for the same reason.

Smoking only two-thirds of your cigarette – most of the poison lurks in the butt.

Becoming a conscious smoker. Count how many you smoke each day – it may shock you to discover that it is more than you think – and try avoiding some of the occasions when you know you are particularly tempted to smoke.

Buying a brand which sells packets of ten and buying only one packet at a time.

Asking your doctor for a prescription for Nicorette, a chewing gum containing a harmless amount of nicotine which you pop in your mouth every time you want a cigarette.

Asking every ex-smoker how they did it.

[16]

Doing it your way

You may be opening this book for the first time at this chapter, or you may have skipped from reading about a cancer on which you wanted particular information to this point because you have cancer. Now you want to know what *you* can do for yourself.

Up to now we have considered only the orthodox medical treatments you can expect to receive for the various cancers. An inherent passivity is implied by the words 'expect' and 'receive' – they suggest that treatment is something decided for you by an expert. You may be invited to ask questions, or even discuss options, but ultimately it is the doctor who knows best about the medical implications and consequences, and he or she will advise you accordingly. Obviously, you can decide not to take the advice and either seek a second opinion or refuse the treatment.

These are your rights, though they are sometimes difficult to insist upon when you are feeling ill, frightened and vulnerable. Chapter 17 discusses (among other things) ways of improving communication between you and your doctor so that together you can reach a better understanding of your personal as well as medical needs.

HOLISTIC MEDICINE

Let us now consider some different approaches to cancer, other ways of dealing with your illness. Broadly speaking, these are all the therapies and activities that come within the spectrum of 'complementary' – a term used these days in preference to 'alternative', which suggests either opposition or 'fringe', as some hostile doctors still persist in calling it. They may be traditional healing arts like acupuncture, herbalism or the laying on of hands (faith healing); they could be modern versions of meditation; they could be a special diet, a new exercise routine, a creative pastime like music or art – indeed, anything which engages the whole of you, not just the disease and the symptoms it is producing in your body.

The range and choice is huge, enough to satisfy our many and various individual preferences. Some are things you can learn and do for yourself; others are ongoing treatments which need to be prescribed and monitored as carefully as any orthodox treatment. All are gentle therapies in the healing, caring sense of the word rather than aggressive treatments to fight a disease. They do not promise cure – but then that is a promise no one can honestly make, not even the most brilliant doctor in the world. They do, however, very often provide physical relief, emotional solace, and above all a strong sense that you are doing something positive for yourself. They make you feel involved with your illness and, to some degree, in charge. You are no longer a helpless victim. You are right there in the centre of your being, using your mind and your spirit to overcome your illness. Some are therapies of which humankind has been availing itself since the beginning of history, but the fact that they are of long standing does not mean they have outworn their usefulness. They work with the body, not against it; in the mind, not outside it.

Essentially, this is what is meant by holistic medicine – 'whole-person medicine', as Dr Patrick Pietroni calls it. Pietroni is a pioneering GP who, some years ago, with a few like-minded doctors, founded the British Holistic Medical Association in an attempt to bring together all the healing arts and their practitioners. These are doctors who have recognised that they do not have all the answers for every disease, and in particular not for something as unpredictable and devious as cancer.

Patrick Pietroni practises what he preaches. He runs a GP practice which combines the two streams of medicine. Various complementary practitioners have consulting rooms in his central London health centre and each patient is assessed by all the members of the practice before it is decided, with the patient, who should take special responsibility for their treatment. Clearly this is a matter for flexible thinking and it is kept under constant review, so that the patient may move from one therapist to another as need dictates.

There is another GP practice run along similar lines in Southampton, and a growing number of family doctors are trained practitioners in one or other of the complementary therapies; homeopathy, acupuncture and hypnotherapy are among the more usual ones. There are now many more family doctors who will voluntarily send a patient they cannot cure either to a colleague who has acquired one of these skills or directly to a non-medical complementary practitioner.

Hospital doctors are not, in the main, so open-minded. They have been trained in battle tactics to 'fight', and 'destroy' and 'conquer' disease. The military terminology is intentional. Think how common is the use of aggressive, bellicose language to describe 'the war on cancer', even by kindly, well-meaning people who devote their lives to trying to relieve people's suffering. Consultants can also feel strongly possessive about their patients and the disease they have. They tend to talk about 'my patients' and 'I'm not allowing that sort of person on my ward' — say, a faith healer or a volunteer from a support group. If a patient admits to trying something alternative, they can damn with faint praise — 'I suppose it can't do you any harm, even if it does you no good' — or be crushingly contemptuous — 'Well, of course, if you're going to believe that rubbish . . .' Is it any wonder that some of their 'cases' (should it be casualties?) turn away for ever, hurt and angry, and thereby perhaps miss out on some of the positive benefits of modern medicine.

'Hack, burn and poison. That was all they could offer me. Cancer to me was like having a voodoo put upon me. Everything that happened to me in an orthodox situation led from one stress to greater stress. It was horrendous. Basically, I was infantilised. Patently they didn't give a damn about me.'

The woman who said this had been particularly unlucky, happening to fall into an uncaring system which had pushed her from one cold, brusque doctor to another; orders were given – 'you'll have a mastectomy tomorrow' – but nothing was explained; her natural terror that she was about to repeat her mother's story had been ignored. (Her mother had died of metastatic cancer six weeks after finding a tiny primary tumour in her breast.)

But change is afoot – and in some of the most traditional, entrenched seats of medical learning. Advanced thinkers like Professor Karol Sikora, for instance, at the Hammersmith Hospital in London, are beginning to appreciate the potential psychological benefits of complementary therapies and to realise that they can be more than just palliatives to keep patients with chronic cancer happy. Sikora sees them as an essential and positive part of the adjuvant therapy that patients will need to help them endure some of the latest developments in primary cancer treatments. In the new cancer centre which is being planned for Hammersmith he intends to have a team of complementary therapists working alongside his oncologists. A proponent of 'magic bullet' therapy, the seek-and-destroy-cancer-cells drug which is still in the laboratory stage, he was quoted in an interview for *The Independent*:[1]

> Any advances are going to require even more intensive high-technology medicine than we have now and that's going to be even more frightening for patients. If we agree the best chance of survival is to get through treatment, alternative therapies that help people cope can actually be life-saving.

At the Royal Marsden Hospital, also in London, Richard Wells, an oncology nurse in charge of rehabilitation, has introduced therapeutic massage, aromatherapy, visualisation and relaxation. Patients can also have any diet they like – including, for instance, the Bristol diet from the Bristol Cancer Help Centre or the controversial, but for some people said to be extraordinarily successful, Gerson diet. (Beata Bishop's *A Time to Heal* is an inspiring account of how it cured her cancer, and changed her life.)

'Our service is for all patients,' says Richard Wells, 'whether they be in remission or in continuing illness. We base it on two premises: one, if it's good for the patient, it's good, no matter what anyone says, so if they want it they should have it; and two, our main aim is the optimum restoration of our patients to ensure an ongoing quality of life. It's wonderful to see someone who is going through a tough time with their treatment, or maybe is dying, look and feel better, even if it is only momentarily.'

He is shortly about to introduce art and drama therapy because he believes that these are ways 'we can help patients come to terms with their cancer and also to express what they're feeling'. When he thinks the time is ripe to introduce a new therapy, he writes a rationale for it which he circulates to the whole caring team, paramedics and social workers as well as nurses and doctors, because he wants everyone to be aware and involved with what is going on. Any obstacles he might have encountered at the beginning have dissolved in the face of the obvious benefits that the patients are enjoying. The staff are also warmly encouraged to use the service. Caring for cancer patients is emotionally draining, and they too need regular doses of TLC – tender loving care – to help them continue.

Hippocrates, venerated as the founder of the medical profession, would have been delighted by this emergent *rapprochement* between old and new healing arts. He was entirely holistic in his approach, believing that health was a matter of being in harmony with nature. When disease attacked the body this was an indication that the balance had been upset and that it must be restored by whatever natural means seemed most appropriate: diet, exercise, rest, herbal potions, occasionally surgery, and sometimes nothing. In those days – *c.* 400 BC – it was considered more ethical for the doctor to tell the patient frankly if he felt he could do no more, and send him home. About cancer specifically, Hippocrates wrote in his Aphorisms: 'it is better to give no treatment in cases of hidden cancer; treatment causes speedy death but to omit treatment is to prolong life.' Clearly he could not have envisaged the amazing advances in knowledge and modern technology that have completely transformed some spheres of medical treatment, but no doubt if he were here today he would continue to maintain that there comes a time in a patient's life when the treatment has to stop. Some doctors find this hard to accept.

The complementary practitioners have not changed their views about the value of their therapies – after all why should they? – but they have shifted position slightly. They are less inclined now to assert their superiority in the somewhat self-righteous tones reminiscent of old-fashioned Fabians preaching the moral virtues of socialism.

A new realism has entered their ranks. They are concerned about charlatans sailing under their flag and they realise that it matters for their therapists to be accredited and approved according to standard criteria, especially if they are ever to become part of the NHS total spectrum of health care, which is where we would want them to be. At the moment most clients have to find the money for the therapist's fees out of their own pockets, and they cannot always be certain that they are paying for the services of a *bona fide* practitioner. Of course there are bad doctors too, and it is widely recognised that the mechanism for making complaints and·obtaining compensation in the NHS is creaking and inadequate, but at least it exists. A client with a grievance against a complementary practitioner has little or no redress. The leading professional associations of the various therapies are well aware of this and realise how much it exposes them to attack from conventional medical quarters. They are far from complacent; they have tightened up on their rules for membership and are keeping a more vigilant eye on examinations and qualifications. A weekend course in acupuncture, for example, is inadequate and unfair, both to the unsuspecting client and to other members of the speciality, many of whom will have studied at least as long as doctors for their qualifications.

Finding out what suits you best can take time; you will need to sample and test, and listen to what friends and other cancer survivors tell you has helped them. The Bristol Cancer Help Centre has been a wonderful starting point for many people, and even if you cannot afford their residential fees, they have tapes and books which you can try at home. Ten years ago they were alone in the field. Now there are several other such places and a wealth of possible therapies to choose from, which is why I have not attempted to describe any in this chapter. (See Resources for an extensive list of addresses and books.)

THE PRUDENT DIET AND SENSIBLE EXERCISE

In 1960 the World Health Organisation estimated that approximately 60 to 70 per cent of cancers were environmentally induced. Today that estimate has rise to 80 per cent, of which 35 per cent are attributed to diet.[2] In part this is because of what we choose to eat – specifically, too much fat and too little fresh fruit, vegetables and other foods with a high fibre, vitamin and mineral content. It may also be due to factors beyond our control. There has recently been a series of appalling revelations about food contamination and adulteration which makes one seriously question what chance there is of escaping cancer by ingestion. But there are positive things we can do for ourselves.

We have already discussed diet in relation to breast cancer (see pages 16–17), where it seems there could be a special connection with a high-fat diet. In this country we eat 20 per cent more saturated fat than we should. Too many of us are also seriously overweight, large enough to be deemed obese in medical terms. Twice as many women as men fall into this category.

It will improve your looks, as well as your health in general, to adopt what the Americans call the Prudent Diet. It really is not that difficult, and once you have re-educated your palate you will also find it enjoyable. It means cutting down on your consumption of red meat, dairy products, sugar, and refined flour and grain products, substituting for them chicken, white meats and fish plus plenty of fresh vegetables, fruit and whole-grain foods; these are rich in proteins, minerals, vitamins and the fibre to stimulate daily bowel action. If you combine a good diet with sufficient regular exercise which is reasonably vigorous but is not overdone and remains pleasurable, you will have dramatically improved your lifestyle, and your chances of living into a healthy old age. Exercise is said to reduce the risk of breast cancer and cancers of the reproductive system.

If you have cancer now, you may want to make more radical changes to your diet. BACUP (see Resources) has a free booklet on diet for cancer patients, and many hospitals have their own diet sheets. It is difficult to say how much difference a special (complementary) diet makes to the course of cancer, but if it makes you feel better, that is as good a reason as any for following it. However, these diets are not for everyone; they require a lot of self-discipline and some people lose weight and feel very ill on them. No one should feel discouraged if they find that after all they cannot stick to them. Doctors are concerned that complementary practitioners sometimes make their patients feel that the diet will cure them. Then, when it doesn't, they feel even sicker, and sad and angry too.

Keep an eye on your drinking. Recent studies have thrown up quite an alarming statistical link between alcohol consumption and breast cancer. Even consuming as few as nine units a week increases your risk by 30 per cent, and higher levels can take it up to 60 per cent. (A unit is equivalent to a glass of wine, a measure of spirits, or half a pint of beer or cider.)

SUPPORT GROUPS

Many support groups are started by cancer patients when they leave hospital and realise they need to talk to someone who has shared something of their experience. A few doctors see the value of these self-help groups and will give their assistance and time to keep them flourishing but on the whole they are patient-led. This can have disadvantages as well as benefits, because it can be deeply upsetting if members of the group die. Usually the groups that function most successfully are run by ex-patients who have had some training in counselling and group dynamics. A sympathetic medical person who can be called on at times of crisis to give calm, professional help is invaluable.

CancerLink is a national voluntary organisation which liaises between such groups (more than 300 of them). It also offers specialised training for members, and help and advice to people who want to start a group in their area. New Approaches to Cancer (ANAC) does the same thing for groups which are more inclined to the complementary field. (Addresses in Resources.)

Everyone has to find their own way of coping with cancer. Talking about cancer with fellow-sufferers, reading up on the subject, or taking up some new constructive activity are all ways people choose. Each of us has to find the one that is right for our circumstances and our temperament. A few years ago, cancer care as opposed to cancer treatment was practically unknown. Today, there are many splendid organisations and individuals who are ready to extend that helping hand. There is sure to be one to suit you among those listed at the back of this book.

[17]

Being your own woman

Knowledge gives us power. A sense of self-esteem, feeling valued and loved, gives us strength. Power and strength are what we need most when we enter a life-threatening crisis, so that we may keep a hold on ourselves and the situation. We may not be able to control it entirely, but we do want to have some understanding of what is happening to us.

A verdict of cancer is such a crisis. For the many thousands of people who are having to confront it now – today, as you read these words – it is probably the most terrifying moment in their lives, but too often the circumstances in which they find themselves when that moment occurs drain away their defences. They feel weak and powerless. They literally do not know what to say, who to ask or where to turn. Sadly, I have heard these words so many times: 'Nobody told me anything' or 'He just said, "cancer, you've got cancer" and then walked away.'

Possibly, their memory is at fault. The very word 'cancer' is enough to drive everything else out of their mind. 'I felt it was a death sentence.' But others, who have been shattered by the same blow, remember also the kindness and warmth that flowed out to them: perhaps from the doctor squeezing their hand as he gave them the diagnosis, or the nurse who put her arms round them in a gentle, wordless hug.

Strength is restored by such simple gestures; they demonstrate a sense of common humanity, and a willingess to share in the pain and grief and to help as much as possible. The cancer patient will need a lot of this support as she goes through her treatments and starts putting her life together again.

But where is the power to come from? Cancer, as we have seen, is a baffling and unpredictable disease. Even the doctors who have worked longest and hardest in the field admit that they are constantly surprised by the unexpected quirks and turns of the disease. The quest for a cancer cure, by the turn of the century if possible, has taken on the mythical aura of the Holy Grail quest. There are armies of researchers spending millions of our money every year, seeking the knowledge we all want, and still the doctors do not have certain answers to some of the most basic questions their patients ask them: 'Can you cure me?' 'Is this fatal?' 'How long have I got?' 'Will this treatment work?' 'Will the cancer come back?'

It is really not fair to ask doctors questions they cannot truthfully answer – or only partially – but when your body and your life are in the balance, fairness is about the last thing on your mind. Most doctors know enough to know how little they know. Many of them find it hard to admit this, because they think it is tantamount to a confession of failure. They believe they are letting themselves down and needlessly destroying their patients' trust in them, so very often they are tempted to appear overconfident.

'Nothing to worry about', they affirm breezily, or: 'We'll soon have that out, and you'll be good as new' – phrases which may pass for positive and reassuring at the time, at least to the speaker, but when the patient starts mulling them over or things do not proceed as smoothly as promised, they begin to assume ominous overtones. 'He's only saying that because he knows it's hopeless', is a common over-reaction. Being told not to worry when cancer is suspected is rather like being told not to be afraid of walking through an inner-city underpass at night. You can't be certain that there is somebody or something hostile lurking down there, out to get you, but it's sure as hell a real possibility, enough to make you sweat with fear. The less you know, the more you fear. Therefore, to make light of your anxieties is to imply that you are making a fuss about nothing, and that is insulting to anyone's intelligence.

Anyone who is being treated for 'a nasty little lump' knows in their heart that cancer is a reality. They may want to deny it, because for them that happens to be the best way they have of coping with their disease, but this does not mean that their concerns should be treated anything less than seriously. They may even have developed a tacit understanding with their doctor that the word 'cancer' is not to be mentioned, and their need for this self-protective blocking mechanism should be understood and respected. This, incidentally, is an example of good communication, because it shows that the doctor is listening to what the patient is *not* telling him, and responding appropriately.

But there will be others who will want to know as much as the doctor can tell them, and more. The insatiable questioner who is never satisfied with the answers she is given is often branded by doctors as neurotic, a tiresome troublemaker. Skilled communicators suggest that the problem may not be as one-sided as it looks. Although words are being exchanged in great abundance, is either side actually hearing what the other is saying? And if not, why not? A woman who feels she is being patronised or getting a brush-off, or suspects that a crucial piece of information is being withheld from her, is – understandably – likely to become more demanding and 'difficult' the more she feels she is not being treated with respect. The amenable patient who is 'compliant to treatment', as doctors are wont to say approvingly, may be equally unhappy and fearful but less able to articulate her concerns.

'NOW TELL ME WHAT YOU KNOW . . .'

This is the way one doctor often starts his consultation. By placing himself at the patient's disposal and inviting her to open herself out to him, he has immediately given her the positive encouragement she needs to voice her problems and to ask the questions she might otherwise have thought 'too important for a busy doctor to waste time on'. Meanwhile, by giving her the initiative he has the space he needs to collect his thoughts and think out his responses. Once a dialogue has been opened in this informal, friendly way, it can ebb and flow, pause and be picked up again, and finally cease – but always with the understanding that it can be resumed on another occasion.

Equality is a difficult notion to sustain in the patient-doctor relationship because so much is weighted in favour of the doctor. Knowledge, expertise, experience and health are all his. The patient has only her sense of self, her personal biography and her lifetime collection of values. Even if she doesn't feel ill, she feels physically and psychologically under threat. The doctor is operating in his domain. He has a staff working for him and he knows what is going to happen next because he is in charge. The patient, on the other hand, is a scared newcomer entering an alien institution. She has no idea what goes on in it, or what to expect.

The only way that some kind of balance can be brought into this relationship is by the doctor offering to share his power. Volunteering information is the first step. In a good interaction a sensitive doctor will quickly pick up how much his patient wants to know about her illness and to what extent she wants to be involved in her treatment. Unfortunately not all doctors are good communicators, and neither are all patients.

LETTING THE DOCTOR KNOW WHAT YOU WANT TO KNOW

Doctors tend to assume that they know what is best for the patient. Sometimes patients agree with them. They find the whole idea of discussing their treatment distasteful and bewildering. They believe that it is the doctor's job to make these decisions for them. That is what he has been trained to do, and they feel quite happy about leaving it all to him. If that is how you feel, then you will have no difficulty in saying so right at the beginning, but remember: you can always change your mind at any time.

Most patients, however, do want to know what to expect, at least as much as the doctor can honestly tell them. If you are reading this book, you are probably one of them. You are probably also the sort of person who would like to be involved in making decisions about your treatment, particularly if you know that there are choices available. Many patients do not, for one simple reason: they have not been told. Paternalistic doctors justify this action by saying that they are removing a cruel burden from their shoulders. It is asking too much, they say, to expect people to make treatment decisions on top of coping with the fact of their cancer. But have they asked the patient what she would like? Invariably not.

If you want to be a fully informed and participating, grown-up, equal partner with your doctor in your healing enterprise – 'joint adventurers in a common cause' as the late Paul Ramsey, the American medical ethicist, put it – then you may have to say so, firmly and clearly, right at the start.[1] Doctors who are equally mature will respond positively because they find it makes their own job so much easier. There are studies to show that patients who are well informed about their disease and know what to expect during treatment recover faster and often do better long-term as well. But there will always be some doctors who find it very difficult to communicate with their patients at any level. It may be because they have problems handling their own emotions, in which case they are not going to do any better at helping you with yours. Or it could be a matter of simple chemistry. You are just not each other's sort of person, and never will be.

Whatever the reason for the clash, don't struggle on your own or suffer in silence. If the doctor can't see that a third person is needed to step in between you, or won't suggest someone from his team, you will have to draw on your own resources. Try always to have your partner, a friend or close relative accompany you when you talk to the doctor. If you feel lonely and isolated, or have no one close to you in whom you want to confide, try asking one of the information sources listed at the end of the book to put you in touch with a counsellor or support group.

MAKING INFORMED DECISIONS

In 1986 an important consensus conference on breast cancer was held by the King's Fund. Its purpose was to issue a policy statement for the future treatment of breast cancer in all its aspects, based on presentations by the leading breast cancer specialists. One of the adjudicating panel's major recommendations was that women who wished to be involved in treatment decisions should be helped and encouraged in every way to participate. Counselling, it recommended, should be available at all stages of treatment, and women should be given time to consider their options.[2]

More recently, the booklet on breast cancer screening which has been sent out to every GP in the country states quite unequivocally:

> The benefits and disadvantages of all procedures, whether surgery, radiotherapy, hormonal therapy, or chemotherapy, should be fully discussed with the woman. Her personal preference for a particular treatment option will be determined by many variables. Clinical information about survival and recurrence rates will be involved, together with a consideration of her personal circumstances.[3]

So it's official: women must be informed about the options open to them, and their preferences must be taken into consideration when it comes to deciding on treatment. Implicitly, what is being said is that doctors must enlist their patients' co-operation in their treatment and ask for their consent. Perhaps you think this happens anyway. And what is so special about breast cancer? you may ask. Anyway, isn't informed consent a legal requirement?

People tend to reel back in astonishment when they hear that doctors aren't legally obliged to tell you anything, and they can even tell you a lie if, in their opinion, the truth might do you harm. The reason for emphasising the need for choice to be made available to women with breast cancer is because there is no consensus opinion on *the* invariable best treatment for this particular disease. On occasions when there is no room for doubt – only one treatment will do – the doctor must obviously make this plain to the patient. These two statements make it clear, however, that doctors do have a strong moral obligation to respond to a woman's request for information. One of these days – and it will be sooner rather than later – that obligation will be tested in court.

In some instances, the informing process may take a considerable amount of time. The treatments, as we have seen, can be complicated to explain to a non-medical person, but that is not an insuperable obstacle. If the language is plain English and the information is delivered empathetically – and repeated, if necessary, several times for it to sink in – then most women will understand soon enough what they need to know for their personal future. No one should imagine, however, that this is going to be an easy time for anyone. The case for more nurse counsellors is overwhelming.

'Though I state this calmly now, the fact that I had a choice completely threw me at the time. We thought we were going to the specialist to be told. I had heard about "informed consent", and here we were being asked to give it. In hindsight, however, having been given the reassurance that my long-term survival rate would not be affected by our decision, to be offered a choice was very important to me as indeed it was my body that was being discussed.'[4]

To reassure research-orientated doctors who find it difficult to accept any innovative practice unless it has been validated by a rigorous controlled study, there is now strong evidence to show that women offered the opportunity to choose their own treatment for breast cancer adapt better psychologically afterwards.[5,6] Women will probably not be surprised by these conclusions.

CLINICAL TRIALS

Breast cancer has been the subject of more studies than most other cancers. The controversy about treatments, the multiple manifestations of the disease, and the uncertainty about its method of dissemination have all been good reasons for a seemingly inexhaustible plethora of randomised clinical trials. Some would say – doctors among them – that too many of these trials have been inexcusably repetitive. It is true that small but statistically significant results are beginning to emerge which have been discussed in earlier chapters in this book, and for that we must be grateful.

This gratitude should, however, be tempered by sadness when we consider the price that has been paid by our sisters to achieve those results. Untold thousands of anonymous women have lent their bodies to these trials. Without their participation the learned doctors who devised and ran the trials, and reaped honours for so doing, would not now be holding important conferences all over the world to debate the results.

Many of the women who made those results possible will be dead now, and perhaps it is better that they will never know how their trust had been betrayed. They didn't know that when the doctor told them this was the treatment he felt was best for them, it was untrue. He did not know, and it was because he did not know, that he had entered them into a study where a computer randomly selected them for one or the other of the treatments on trial. There is nothing wrong with this procedure – randomisation ensures impartiality – but these women were deprived of the chance to make a competent, informed decision about their treatment. They were not treated as adult, rational persons, capable of making up their own minds. Many of these same women would willingly have given their consent to inclusion in the trial, and accepted the randomising procedure, had they only been asked. It is a characteristic of cancer patients to want to take any chance for themselves while at the same time hoping their participation will help future generations.

Since I have already written a detailed critique of the ethics of informed consent and randomised clinical trials (see Further Reading) I will make only the following points here. Any woman who enters hospital for treatment of any kind, for cancer or any other condition, is entitled to ask whether she is being considered for entry into a randomised controlled trial. If she is, she should be fully informed about the trial, its aims and objectives, what the treatment options are, how she will be selected, and what are the anticipated risks and benefits. She has the right to withdraw from the trial at any point.

Doctors like to emphasise that these trials, on the whole, are well conceived and supervised so that patients who are entered into them can be assured of a high standard of care and follow-up. But then isn't that what we expect anyway, in or out of a trial?

Evelyn Thomas is a breast cancer patient and an exceptionally courageous and determined woman. She was first treated for her cancer in 1982 and several years later, after reading a newspaper article, realised she must have participated in the trial it described. After a long saga of rebuffs, unanswered letters and unsatisfactory meetings, verging at times on the Kafkaesque, which would have defeated most healthier people — and by now Evelyn had advanced cancer — she finally forced her doctors to admit that they had entered her into two trials without her consent. Throughout she has always behaved with dignity and restraint. Her one hope is that her struggle will have been all worthwhile if it never happens again to anyone. She reminds us all that 'patients are the people whom doctors trust to teach and care for their children, cook their food, police their streets and pay their salaries. It is only in hospital and by doctors that we are considered incapable of making responsible choices: such assumptions cause great resentment.'[7]

LIFE AFTER CANCER – TESTIMONIES

Cancer is a unique experience for each person who has it. Those of us who have not been through it can probably never totally comprehend its meaning, but the breath of cancer touches us all. We will all know people in our lives who have cancer, had it, or have been cured of it, and some of them will be very dear and close to us.

Life will never be the same again, grieves the woman looking down at the flattened lopsided plane of her chest. She is right and it is true for her, as it is true for everyone in different ways at different times. Life changes all the time. Life changes us, and our life changes the lives of others. We cannot escape our human condition, and the more deeply we are committed to living and loving in all its aspects – people, work, politics, pleasures: all that absorbs and fulfils us – the more vulnerable we are to loss. Sickness, accidents and death threaten us all. They are the price we pay for living, and sooner or later the toll will be exacted from each and every one of us.

Cancer is an exceptionally cruel demand, yet in some ways it can be seen as a gift. Unlike the sudden death which comes from an accident or a heart attack or the living death of a stroke or senile dementia, cancer usually offers a breathing space, and sometimes a new life. People often say that it has made them rethink their priorities and helped them to acquire a more meaningful perspective.

No one can speak more profoundly about cancer than the cancer survivor. Many of them do so much more than survive. They thrive and accomplish extraordinary things. This book ends with some of their words.

'Saying that you're alive is not enough. Living with it is the real test.' (Judith)

'I've wound down my life and now I'm enjoying every day I've got.' (Jo)

'I'm going to go on living until I die.' (Betty)

Chapter references

1 BOSOM THOUGHTS

1. James Laver, *Modesty in Dress: an Inquiry into the Fundamentals of Fashion*, William Heinemann, 1969.

2 WHY DO WOMEN GET BREAST CANCER?

1. Cancer Research Campaign, *Facts on Cancer* (regularly updated Factsheets on cancer statistics. Source of all British cancer statistics quoted throughout this book).

2. Olivia Timbs and Lorraine Fraser, 'Medical Briefing', *The Times*, 2 October 1984.

3. Ellen Grant, *The Bitter Pill*, pp. 104–05, Corgi, 1985.

4. C. R. Kay and P. C. Hannaford, 'Breast Cancer and the Pill – a Further Report from the Royal College of General Practitioners' Oral Contraception Study', *British Journal of Cancer*, vol. 58 (1988), pp. 675–80.

5. Clair Chilvers, Dr K. McPherson, Professor J. Peto, Professor M. C. Pike and Professor M. P. Vessey, 'Oral Contraceptive Use and Breast Cancer Risk in Young Women', *The Lancet*, 6 May 1989, pp. 973–82.

6. 'Oral Contraceptives and Neoplasia', editorial, *The Lancet*, 22 October 1983.

7. Daniel R. Mishell, 'Contraception', *New England Journal of Medicine*, vol. 320, no. 12 (1989), pp. 777–87.

8. Malcolm Whitehead, 'Hormone Replacement Therapy as Preventative Medicine', paper given at conference on *Modern Approaches to Health Promotion for the Well Woman – and Man*, Middlesex Hospital, 1 July 1988.

9. S. Greer and T. Morris, 'Psychological Attributes of Women who Develop Breast Cancer: A Controlled Study', *Journal of Psychosomatic Research*, 19, pp. 147–53.

4. I'VE GOT A LUMP IN MY BREAST

1. Jennifer Hughes, *Cancer & Emotion*, pp. 35–36, John Wiley, 1987.

5 SCREENING COULD SAVE YOUR LIFE

1. J. Chamberlain *et al.*, 'First Results on Mortality Reduction in the UK Trial of Early Detection of Breast Cancer', *The Lancet*, 20 August 1988, pp. 411–16.

2. Working group chaired by Professor Sir Patrick Forrest, *Breast Cancer Screening*, HMSO, 1986.

3. Petr Skrabanek, 'False Premises and False Promises of Breast Cancer Screening', *The Lancet*, 10 August 1985, pp. 316–19.

4. Joan Austoker and John Humphreys, *Breast Cancer Screening*, p. 21, Oxford Medical Publications, 1988.

5. Principles of screening first formulated in 1968 by Wilson and Jungner for the World Health Organisation.

6. E. G. Knox, 'Evaluation of a Proposed Breast Cancer Screening Regimen', *British Journal of Medicine*, vol. 297, 10 September 1988, pp. 650–54.

7 IS YOUR OPERATION REALLY NECESSARY?

1. Joyce Hemlow (ed.), *Fanny Burney: The Journal and Letters*, vol. VI, Letter 595, pp. 595–615, Oxford University Press, 1972.

2. Sir Geoffrey Keynes, 'A Historical Perspective', Foreword to *Primary Management of Breast Cancer: Alternatives to Mastectomy*, ed. Jeffrey S. Tobias and Michael J. Peckham, Edward Arnold, 1985.

3. J. Morris, G. T. Royle and I. Taylor, 'Changes in the Surgical Management of Early Breast Cancer in England', *Journal of the Royal Society of Medicine*, vol. 82, January 1989, pp. 12–14.

4. Bernard Fisher *et al.*, 'Five-Year Results of a Randomized Clinical Trial comparing Total Mastectomy and Segmental Mastectomy with or without Radiation in the Treatment of Breast Cancer',

New England Journal of Medicine, vol. 312, 14 March 1985, pp. 665–73. Also in same issue, pp. 674–81, paper on 'Ten-Year Results' of similar trial, also by Bernard Fisher *et al*. And most recently, the 'Eight-Year Results' of the first trial mentioned have been published in the *New England Journal of Medicine*, vol. 320, 30 March 1989, pp. 822–28. The findings are consistent: namely, that there is no difference in survival outcome between lumpectomy and mastectomy. Irradiation following lumpectomy reduces the probability of local recurrence.

8 CONSERVATION OR RECONSTRUCTION

1. See chapter 7, note 3.
2. Leslie E. Botnick, Jay R. Harris and Samuel Hellman, 'Experience with Breast Conserving Approaches at the Joint Center for Radiation Therapy, Boston', in *Primary Management of Breast Cancer: Alternatives to Mastectomy*, ed. Jeffrey S. Tobias and Michael J. Peckham, Edward Arnold, 1985.
3. Audre Lorde, *The Cancer Journals*, Sheba Feminist Publishers, 1980.
4. R. Glynn Owens, J. J. Ashcroft, P. D. Slade and S. J. Leinster, 'Psychological Effects of the Offer of Breast Reconstruction following Mastectomy', Proceedings of the Second and Third meetings of the British Psychosocial and Oncology Group London and Leicester, 1985 and 1986. *Psychosocial Oncology*, 1985 and 1986.
5. Carol Brickman, 'Surviving Every Woman's Nightmare', *The Times*, 23 September 1985.
6. C. Dean, U. Chetty and A. P. M. Forrest, 'Effects of Immediate Breast Reconstruction on Psychosocial Morbidity after Mastectomy', *The Lancet*, 1983 i, pp. 459–62.

9 WHAT ELSE CAN THEY DO?

1. *New England Journal of Medicine*, vol. 320, 23 February 1989, pp. 473–96.
2. W. L. McGuire, 'Adjuvant Therapy of Node Negative Breast Cancer', editorial, ibid., pp. 525–27.
3. V. T. De Vita, 'Breast Cancer Therapy: Exercising all our Options', editorial, ibid., pp. 527–29.
4. Early Breast Cancer Trialists' Collaborative Group, 'Effects of

Adjuvant Tamoxifen and of Cytotoxic Therapy on Mortality in
Early Breast Cancer: an Overview of 61 Randomized Trials among
28,896 Women', *New England Journal of Medicine*, vol. 319, pp.
1681–92.

5. W. L. McGuire, 'Adjuvant Therapy . . .'. See note 2.

6. *New England Journal of Medicine*, vol. 320.

7. 'Adjuvant Systemic Treatment for Breast Cancer Meta-ana-
lysed', editorial in *The Lancet*, 14 January 1989, pp. 80–81.

11 HELP IS THERE

1. Laura Pendleton and Alwyn Smith, 'Provision of Breast
Prostheses', *Nursing Times*, 4 June 1986.

12 THE ONE WE NEEDN'T HAVE

1. Petr Skrabanek, 'Cervical Cancer in Nuns and Prostitutes: A
Plea for Scientific Continence', *Journal of Clinical Epidemiology*,
vol. 41, no. 6 (1988), pp. 577–82.

2. 'Is Cervical Laser Therapy Painful?', *The Lancet*, 14 January
1989, p. 83; and subsequent correspondence in ibid., 11 February
1989, p. 335.

3. Jean Robinson, 'Cancer of the Cervix: Occupational Risks of
Husbands and Wives and Possible Preventative Strategies', in *Pre-
Clinical Neoplasia of the Cervix, Proceedings of the Ninth Study
Group of the Royal College of Obstetricians and Gynaecologists*,
ed. J. A. Jordan, F. Sharp and A. Singer, London, 1982, pp. 11–27.

4. Tina Posner and Martin Vessey, letter to *The Lancet*, 4 March
1989, pp. 494–95.

13 THE SECRET ENEMY

1. Cancer and Steroid Hormone Study of the Centers for Disease
Control and the National Institute of Child Health and Human
Development, 'The Reduction in Risk of Ovarian Cancer Associated
with Oral Contraceptive Use', *New England Journal of Medicine*,
vol. 316 (1987), pp. 650–55.

2. 'Oral Contraceptive Use and the Risk of Endometrial Cancer',
Journal of the American Medical Association, vol. 249 (1983), pp.
1600–04.

3. Data presented at St Bartholomew's Hospital, 11 October 1988.

4. Ian Jacobs, David Oram *et al.*, 'Multimodal Approach to Screening for Ovarian Cancer', *The Lancet*, 6 February 1988, pp. 268–71.

5. M. A. Capone, K. S. Westie and R. S. Good, 'Enhancing Sexual Rehabilitation of the Gynecologic Cancer Patient: A Counseling Treatment Model and Outcome', in *Body Image, Self-Esteem and Sexuality in Cancer Patients*, ed. Vaeth, 2nd edn, Karger, Basel, 1986, pp. 139–47.

14 BLACK SPOT

1. The Cancer Research Campaign is focusing its initial effort on six selected cities: London, Edinburgh, Exeter, Nottingham, Southampton and Leicester. These centres have been chosen because of their available records and facilities.

15 THE LAST PUFF

1. S. E. Barton, J. Cuzick, A. Singer *et al.*, 'Effect of Cigarette Smoking on Cervical Epithelial Immunity: A Mechanism for Neoplastic Change?' *The Lancet*, 17 September 1988, pp. 652–54.

2. Liz Batten, 'Smoking Motivations and Cessation Rates: An Analysis of Gender-Based Differences', in *Women in Psychology – Recent Developments in Britain*, ed. Jan Burns and Mathilde de Jong, *Equal Opportunities International*, vol. 5, no. 3/4 (1986), pp. 22–27

3. Ash Women and Smoking Group, '*Women and Smoking: A Handbook for Action*', Health Education Council (now Authority), 1986.

4. Anne Charlton, *Cells, Cancers and Communities*, Stanley Thornes & Hulton, 1988. A teaching pack designed to offer accessible and friendly material to eleven-to-sixteen-year-old schoolchildren.

16 DOING IT YOUR WAY

1. Cathy Read, 'A Positively Better Approach', *The Independent*, 3 January 1989.

2. Nicholas Wells, *Women's Health Today*, Office of Health Economics (November 1987). All figures and information about women's health in this chapter are taken from this book.

17 BEING YOUR OWN WOMAN

1. Paul Ramsey, *The Patient as Person: Explorations in Medical Ethics*, New Haven, 1970.

2. Consensus Statement, King's Fund Forum, 'Treatment of Primary Breast Cancer', British Medical Journal, vol. 293 (1986), pp. 946–47.

3. Joan Austoker and John Humphreys, *Breast Cancer Screening*, p. 33, Oxford Medical Publications, 1988.

4. Written by a patient for article by Gill Day SRN, 'Mastectomy to the ski slopes in six weeks'.

5. R. Glynn Owens, Jennifer J. Ashcroft, S. J. Leinster, Peter D. Slade, 'Informal Decision Analysis with Breast Cancer Patients: An Aid to Psychological Preparation for Surgery', *Journal of Psychosocial Oncology*, vol. 5, no. 2 (1987).

6. Ronald G. Wilson, Alison Hart, P. J. D. K. Dawes, 'Mastectomy or Conservation: the Patient's Choice', *British Journal of Medicine*, vol. 297, 5 November 1988, pp. 1167–69.

7. Evelyn Thomas, 'Review,' *IME Bulletin*, no. 40, July 1988.

Glossary

Abnormal smear a smear result showing an abnormality such as CIN, infection of the cervix, or inflammatory changes.

Adenoma a benign tumour.

Adjuvant auxiliary or additional. Term applied to any therapy which is used as back-up to primary treatment (usually surgery) of primary tumour. Chemotherapy, radiotherapy and hormone therapy can all be used as adjuvants.

Adrenal glands two small organs near the kidneys which are responsible for synthesising and releasing several hormones, primarily catecholamines and steroids.

Aetiology science of the causes of disease.

Axilla armpit; hence **axillary** – relating to the armpit.

Benign medical term for describing a condition which is mild and non-malignant but may require treatment.

Biopsy the surgical removal of a small piece of tissue for laboratory examination by a pathologist to determine whether it is malignant.

Excision biopsy is surgical removal of the whole lump. This may be done under general or local anaesthetic. The laboratory processing and examination take one to two days.

Carcinogen any agent which causes cancer.

Carcinoma a malignant tumour arising in tissue which forms the outer layer of body surface or lining of cavities that open to the body surface. This tissue (called epithelial) includes skin, glands, nerves, breasts and the linings of the respiratory, gastro-intestinal, urinary and genital systems. Carcinomas account for approximately 85 per cent of human cancers.

Carcinoma in situ often also called **pre-invasive carcinoma**. This means that the tumour is contained within its place of origin and has not spread. Removing it at this localised stage offers a very high chance of cure.

Cervix the neck of the uterus (womb) at the top of the vagina.

Chemotherapy the use of one or more anti-cancer (cytotoxic) drugs to destroy cancer cells which have spread from the primary tumour to other parts of the body. If used when cancer is first diagnosed, it is known as **adjuvant chemotherapy** (see **Adjuvant**).

Combination chemotherapy describes the use of several anti-cancer drugs in varying proportions to treat early and advanced cancer. This is based on the principle that their combined use will improve their effectiveness and reduce toxicity.

CIN abbreviation for Cervical Intraepithelial Neoplasia.

Clinical medicine is medical practice based on observed symptoms. Hence **clinical examination** for breast disease is the physical examination of a patient's breast, and **clinical staging** is diagnosing the extent of cancer by analysing the conclusions drawn from the examination.

Colposcopy examination of the cervix through a colposcope, a specially strong microscope placed at the entrance to the vagina which shows up the shapes of cells.

Complementary used to describe treatment outside mainstream cancer therapy, such as homeopathy, herbal medicine. Also called 'alternative'.

Cone biopsy removal of part of the cervix, in the shape of a cone, for tests.

Cyst an accumulation of material, usually fluid, contained in a sac. It is a common non-malignant swelling, only very rarely associated with a cancer.

Cytology microscopic examination of individual or groups of cells.

Cytotoxic anti-cancer. Term applied to the drugs used in chemotherapy.

Dyskaryosis abnormalities seen in the cells taken in the cervical smear. Included in the term **CIN**.

Dysplasia abnormal cells in surface layer of cervix. Included in the term **CIN**, but gives information about the cell abnormalities that can be seen only in the biopsy.

Endocrine or hormone therapy treatment controlling hormone activity in tumours suspected to be hormone-dependent.

Endogenous   growing or originating from within the body.

Endometrium   the inner lining of the womb or uterus.

Epidemiology   science of epidemics and now of disease generally.

Epithelium   a thin layer of lining cells.

Exogenous   growing or originating from outside the body.

Fine-needle aspiration   a technique to differentiate cystic from solid lesions in the breast. A needle is inserted in the lesion and the material drawn out with a syringe. If the material is solid it can be stained and the cells are examined in a laboratory to determine whether they are benign or malignant. This is known as **Fine-needle aspiration cytology**.

Frozen section   small piece of suspect tissue which is cut out (excised) at biopsy, frozen, and sent for immediate pathological examination.

Gamma rays   a type of electromagnetic radiation with wavelengths shorter than those of X-rays. They therefore carry more energy than X-rays and when used for radiotherapy deliver more energy to tumours, except for those X-rays now delivered by a linear accelerator, which has energies of several million volts.

Histology   science of organic tissues; hence **histologic analysis** is examining tissue for changes caused by disease, and **histologic classification** is naming and determining the extent and type of disease.

Hormone   a chemical substance, produced in certain parts of the body, which has a specific effect on the activity of one or more distant organs.

Hormone Replacement Therapy (HRT)   usually refers to treatment of menopausal and post-menopausal women who are given oestrogen by tablet, injection or implant to replace the oestrogen deficiency which is the natural result of the ovaries ceasing to function.

Hysterectomy   removal of the uterus; sometimes cervix, tubes, ovaries are removed too, but often this is not necessary.

Immunology   a scientific study of resistance to infection in humans and animals. Hence **immunological** responses describe ways in which the body defends itself against disease; **immunosuppressive** refers to any agent which prevents these defence mechanisms from operating; and **immunotherapy** is treatment based on principle of supporting or improving the body's natural defence mechanisms.

Implant   artificial substance, usually silicone gel, which is inserted into breast cavity to replace the natural breast.

Inflammatory changes cell damage changes caused by bacteria, viruses, IUD strings, etc., but which are not CIN.

Invasive cells cells that are growing inwards, changing normal body tissue into abnormal, cancerous tissue.

Interval cancer a cancer that is diagnosed because of symptoms within a stated interval after a negative screening test.

Ionising radiation energy emitted as electromagnetic waves, used in radiotherapy and X-ray diagnosis. Must be used with care, as heavy or too many repeated applications can cause cancer.

Laparascopy a minor operation under general anaesthetic in which a fine flexible tube with a telescopic light at the end is inserted through a small cut close to the navel to examine the ovaries. It can also be used to take a small sample of tissue for analysis.

Laparotomy an exploratory abdominal operation.

Laser therapy laser beam used in the treatment of tumours of pre-malignant changes, e.g. of the cervix.

Lesion changes in the functioning or texture of an organ which is caused by disease.

Local recurrence cancer which reappears on site of original tumour. Hence **local therapy** is treatment applied directly to this site.

Lumpectomy the most conservative form of mastectomy, involving removal of malignant tumour only in the breast, together with surrounding tissue.

Lymph colourless fluid from body tissue and organs which resembles blood but has no red corpuscles.

Lymphangioma a benign tumour arising in lymph vessels.

Lymph gland or node small mass of tissue where lymph is purified and lymphocytes are formed. In breast cancer, the condition of the axillary, pectoral and mammary nodes which surround the breast is an important indication for prognosis about the extent of cancer spread.

Lymphocyte a form of **leucocyte**, which is a colourless blood cell also in lymph.

Lymphoedema swelling of the arm caused by fluid which cannot drain away normally because the lymphatic drainage system – i.e. the lymph nodes – have been surgically removed.

Malignant in cancer refers to growths which will spread with potentially fatal results if not removed.

Mamma or mammary gland milk-secreting organ of female mammals; in women called the breast.

Mammography X-ray diagnostic technique specially developed to investigate the breast for cancer cells.

Mastectomy surgical procedure to remove the whole breast.

Medical oncologist doctor who specialises in the medical treatment of cancer, including drugs treatment.

Melanoma type of skin cancer.

Menarche first menstruation.

Menopause period of life, usually between forty-five and fifty-five, when a woman ceases to menstruate, signifying the end of her reproductive life.

Metastasis the process by which malignant cells detach themselves from the primary tumour and establish themselves in distant parts of the body, starting new tumours called **metastases** or **secondaries**.

Morbidity diseased state of organ or tissue.

Neoplasia cancer.

Neoplasm malignant tumour.

Neoplastic of, or relating to, malignant tumours.

Node-positive describes condition of one or more lymph nodes diagnosed as invaded by cancer cells.

Non-invasive cells cancerous cells that have not yet begun to grow inwards.

Nulliparous refers to a woman who has never given birth.

Occult carcinoma a small tumour which is asymptomatic (gives no indication of its presence).

Oncology the study of the causes, development, characteristics and treatment of cancer.

Oopherectomy procedure, either by surgery or radiation, to remove the ovaries, sometimes called **castration**.

Os entrance to the canal through the cervix, from vagina to uterus.

Pathologist specialist in laboratory medicine concerned with identifying the changes in body tissues and organs which cause or are caused by disease.

Pituitary gland, also known as the **hypophysis** A small organ situated at the base of the brain which is responsible for synthesising and releasing at least nine different hormones. Exerts important influence on growth and bodily functions.

Pre-cancerous cells abnormally shaped cells one stage away from being cancer.

Prognosis medical prediction about the development of a disease diagnosed in a patient.

Prolactin hormone, secreted by the pituitary gland, which stimulates the milk flow.

Prophylactic medical action to prevent disease.

Prosthesis artificial part to replace some portion of the human anatomy. Where there has been a mastectomy, the term applies equally to surgical implants and to breast forms, made of various materials, which are put into the empty bra cup.

Punch biopsy very small piece of tissue cut out to be tested.

Quality-adjusted-life-year (QALY) an outcome measure which combines changes in life expectancy as the result of any intervention (life-years gained) with the expected morbidity of quality of life associated with those life-years. It is recognised that comparing the outcomes of different health service interventions only in terms of life-years gained is inappropriate because it is not comparing like with like. Techniques for assessing the relative weight to be given to different types of morbidity are being developed, and quality-adjusted values should be seen as indicative at this stage.

Radiographer professionally trained person who takes radiographs and is involved with other imaging techniques.

Radiologist specialist concerned with the diagnosis of disease by means of imaging techniques.

Radiotherapy treatment of cancer by ionising radiation, which is energy emitted as electromagnetic waves to destroy the malignant cells. In early cancer the aim is to remove all malignancy; in advanced cancer this is no longer possible but it is palliative: i.e. it temporarily lessens the effects of the disease.

Radiotherapist doctor who plans radiotherapy treatment.

Radium radioactive metallic element derived from pitchblende, sometimes used in radiotherapy.

Remission a period of good health occurring after the onset of cancer, it can happen spontaneously or be induced by therapy.

Scan detailed picture of structures inside the body taken with either X-rays (computerised tomography – CT) or using magnetism (magnetic resonance imaging – RMI) or with high-frequency sound waves (ultrasound).

Secondaries recurrence of cancer cells in distant parts of the body after discovery of the primary tumour.

Sensitivity the ability of a test to detect a disease; a test with a sensitivity of 90 per cent will give a positive result in nine out of ten cases of disease present in the screened population.

Smear test   a few flaky cells scraped painlessly off the surface of the cervix and examined under a microscope for abnormal shapes.

Specificity   the ability of a test to exclude people who do not have disease; a test with a specificity of 90 per cent will give a negative result in 900 out of 1,000 non-diseased people who are screened.

Speculum   duck-billed instrument for opening up the vagina and viewing the cervix; some women have their own plastic one.

Squamous cells   cells which cover the surface of the cervix. They are formed into a tough, many-layered sheet, rather like skin.

Steroids   large group of organic compounds including cholesterol, the sex hormones and the D-vitamins. Some steroids can be used as anti-cancer agents.

Survival rate   the proportion of patients with a disease who are alive at a given time after diagnosis (or treatment).

Systemic   refers to the body as a whole system, hence **systemic therapy** is treatment aiming to attack malignancy wherever it may be throughout the body.

Transformation zone   area of metaplasia in which the original squamous cells are replaced by columnar cells.

Tumour   swelling mass of tissue in any part of the body, derived from pre-existing cells, which serves no purpose and grows independently of surrounding tissue. **Benign tumours** remain localised, are usually slow-growing and produce symptoms only when their size interferes with surrounding tissue. **Malignant tumours** have varying rates of growth but eventually, if left untreated, they tend to invade surrounding tissue and spread to other parts of the body.

Ultrasonography   production of a visual image of deep structures of the body by recording the echoes of sound waves directed into the tissues.

Urethra   tube from bladder to exterior of body through which urine is passed.

Vault smear   smear test taken on a woman who has had her cervix and uterus removed and the far end of her vagina sewn up. The smear is taken from this far end because if the cancer were to recur, it would show up here first.

Resources

USEFUL ORGANISATIONS

There are many organisations which offer a wide range of information or support for health professionals, cancer patients and their families and friends. Here are some of the main ones which may be able to give you the information you need or put you in touch with other organisations involved with specific kinds of cancer as well as those offering practical care or counselling. Many will also be able to give you details of help available in your own area.

Action Cancer
129 Marlborough House
Marlborough Park South
Belfast BT9 6HW
Tel: 0232 661081

Provides an early-warning screening service and counselling service.

Action on Smoking and Health (ASH)
5–11 Mortimer Street
London W1N 7RH
Tel: 01-637 9843

Produces and disseminates information to the public and health professionals about the dangers of smoking.

The Association of Sexual and Marital Therapists
PO Box 62,
Sheffield S10 3TS

Will send a list of all the centres where direct treatment of sexual difficulties is available. Also has a list of individual therapists you or your doctor can contact. Send large stamped addressed envelope.

Bristol Cancer Help Centre
Grove House
Cornwallis Grove
Clifton,
Bristol BS8 4PG
Tel: 0272 743216

Runs residential and daytime courses for cancer sufferers. Well known for its diet and other 'gentle' ways of coping with cancer. Provides a list of affiliated groups which is also published in *Turning Point*, its new magazine.

British Association for Counselling (BAC)
37A Sheep Street
Rugby
Warwickshire CV21 3BX
Tel: 0788 78328/9

Refers clients to qualified counsellors in their own area.

The British Association of Cancer United Patients (BACUP)
121/123 Charterhouse Street,
London, EC1M 6AA
Tel: 01-608 1785 (Admin.)
        01-608 1661 (Cancer Infor. Service)
                Freeline (outside London) 0800 181199
        01-608 1036 (Counselling)

Offers information and support to cancer patients and their families and friends. A team of experienced cancer nurses provides detailed information on all aspects of cancer and services available throughout the country. BACUP produces a range of free publications on the main types of cancers and different ways of living and coping with cancer. Also publishes a free newspaper three times a year to which patients, relatives or friends can contribute letters or articles.

Breast Care and Mastectomy Association (BCMA)
26A Harrison Street
London, WC1H 8JG
Tel: 01-837 0908

Offers non-medical advice and practical support over the telephone and can introduce women who have had breast surgery to a volunteer in their own area who has had similar treatment and can share the experience. Produces several free publications and has a video available for loan – *Looking Good* – which features a group of women who have all had breast surgery and shows how they have come to terms with their individual experiences. Particularly good for advice on prostheses and clothes to wear, and where to find them.

BUPA
Women's Screening Unit
Battle Bridge House
300 Gray's Inn Road
London WC1X 8DU
Tel: 01-278 4651
      01-837 6484
      Appointments 01-837 7055

Offers a complete well woman check-up. Also has mobile breast screening units in various regions. Fees and further information on request.

The Jeannie Campbell Breast Cancer Radiotherapy Appeal
29 St Luke's Avenue
Ramsgate
Kent CT11 7JZ
Tel: 0843 596732 & 593193

Provides information on all treatment options for women with breast cancer.

CancerLink
17 Britannia Street
London WC1X 9JN
Tel: 01-833 2451

CancerLink (Scottish Infor. Service)
9 Castle Terrace
Edinburgh EH1 2DP
Tel: 031–228 5557
(Open Mon-Thurs 1–5 p.m. Answering machine other times.)

Provides information and support on all aspects of cancer to people with cancer, their families and friends, and professionals working with them. Acts as a resource centre to cancer support and self-help groups and helps people who set up new groups. Produces various helpful booklets and directories.

Cancer Aftercare and Rehabilitation Society (CARE)
21 Zetland Road
Redland
Bristol BS6 7AH
Tel: 0272 427419

An organisation of cancer patients, relatives and friends who offer help and support. Branches throughout the country.

Cancer Relief Macmillan Fund
15–19 Britten Street
London SW3 3TZ
Tel: 01-351 7811

Office for Scotland
9 Castle Terrace
Edinburgh EH1 2DP
Tel: 031–229 3276

Funds specially trained Macmillan nurses to care for cancer patients in their own home or in hospitals. Also provides financial help for cancer patients in need.

Cancer Research Campaign
2 Carlton House Terrace
London SW1Y 5AR
Tel: 01-930 8972

Produces materials for schools, colleges and the general public on many aspects of cancer and research, including CRC statistical factsheets ('Facts on Cancer'), a breast screening booklet and a leaflet on the early-warning signs for malignant melanoma.

College of Health
18 Victoria Park Square
Bethnal Green
London E2 9PF
Tel: 01-980 6263

Will send a list of specialist NHS breast units and clinics.

Community Health Councils
Find them in your phone book or Yellow Pages.

CRUSE
Cruse House
126 Sheen Road
Richmond
Surrey TW9 1UR
Tel: 01-940 4818/9047

A national organisation for the widowed and their children. Offers a counselling service to help with the emotional difficulties of bereavement and practical advice. There is a network of local branches throughout the country.

CYANA (Cancer You Are Not Alone)
31 Church Road
London E12 6AD
Tel: 01-533 5366 (office hours)
      01-472 8861 (after hours)

The Family Planning Association
27/35 Mortimer Street
London W1N 7RJ
Tel: 01-636 7866 (Mon–Thurs 9.00–5.00; Friday
9.00–4.30; answering machine after hours.)

The Genetic Clinic (Dr Joan Slack)
Royal Free Hospital
Pond Street
London NW3 2QG
Tel: 01–402 4200, ext. 372

Offers screening and advice to women with close relatives who developed breast cancer before the age of fifty.

Health Education Authority
Hamilton House
Mabledon Place
London WC1H 9TX
Tel: 01–631 0930

Publishes a source list of cancer education publications and teaching aids, including a free booklet, *Can You Avoid Cancer?*

The Herpes Association
41 North Road
London N7 9DP
Tel: 01-609 9061 (24 hours)

Hospice Information Service
St Christopher's Hospice
51–59 Lawrie Park Road
Sydenham
London SE26 6DZ
Tel: 01-778 9252

Provides a Directory of Hospice Services including inpatient units, home care support teams and hospital support teams in the UK.

The Hysterectomy Support Group
11 Henryson Road
Brockley
London SE4 1HL
Tel: 01-690 5987

Provides information. There are similar support groups in other parts of the country, often attached to a well woman clinic or set up on a volunteer basis through a hospital.

Imperial Cancer Research Fund
PO Box 123
Lincoln's Inn Fields
London WC2A 3PX
Tel: 01-242 0200

Produces a series of educational publications and videos on various aspects of cancer, including cervical cancer, breast cancer and cancer prevention. Their video *One Woman in Twelve* shows new advances in breast surgery and treatment and demonstrates the value of breast screening.

ICM (The Institute for Complementary Medicine)
21 Portland Place
London W1N 3AF
Tel: 01-636 8543 (office hours, seven days a week)

Provides information about various professional associations in complementary therapy and funds research.

Irish Cancer Society
5 Northumberland Road
Dublin 4
Eire
Tel: Dublin (001) 681855 or Cancer Freefone

Disseminates information on prevention, early detection and continuing care of patients with cancer. The Society funds a night nursing service and a home care service; its rehabilitation programmes include Reach to Recovery, the Colostomy Care Group and the Laryngectomy Association of Ireland.

The Dr Jan de Winter Clinic for Cancer Prevention Advice
6 New Road
Brighton
Sussex BN1 1UF
Tel: 0273–727213 (10.00–4.00)
0323–870500 (after hours)

Marie Curie Cancer Care
28 Belgrave Square
London SW1X 8QG
Tel: 01-235 3325

Runs eleven nursing homes throughout the UK and a community nursing service to give extended care to patients at home.

Marie Stopes House
108 Whitfield Street
London W1P 6BE
Tel: 01-388 0662 (office hours)

Provides cervical smear service, including a cervigram, birth control and sterilisation.

Matthew Manning Centre
39 Abbeygate Street
Bury St Edmunds
Suffolk IP33 1LW
Tel: 0284–69502/752364 (Mon–Fri 9.00–5.30)

Faith healing.

National Society of Non Smokers (QUIT)
40–48 Hanson Street
London W1P 7DE
Tel: 01-636 9103

Offers practical advice to people who want to stop smoking.

New Approaches to Cancer
c/o The Seekers Trust
Addington Park
Maidstone
Kent ME19 5BL
Tel: 0732-848336 (Mon–Fri 9.00–5.00, then answering machine.)

Aims to improve communication between cancer sufferers and those able to help them through holistic therapy; also to take the fear out of cancer by providing information and support. Acts as referral centre and network for more than 300 support groups and individuals.

Patients Association
18 Victoria Park Square
Bethnal Green
London E2 9PF
Tel: 01-981 5676/5695

Provides an advice service for patients independent of government and health professionals. Produces booklets on a range of subjects, including patients' rights and changing your doctor under the NHS.

Scottish Health Education Group (SHEG)
Health Education Centre
Woodburn House
Canaan Lane
Edinburgh EH10 4SG
Tel: 031–447 8044

Information and publications on all aspects of health, including cancer in Scotland. Offers a free publication 'Can You Avoid Cancer?'

Tak Tent
4th Floor, G Block
Western Infirmary
Glasgow G11 6NT
Tel: 041–332 3639

Provides information, support and counselling for cancer patients, relatives and professional staff. A wide range of literature is available. Can provide counselling help in person or by phone. Details of local groups in Glasgow and west/central Scotland can be obtained from Tak Tent.

Tenovus
111 Cathedral Road
Cardiff CF1 9PH
Tel: 0222 42851

Provides a counselling and information service personally or over the phone.

Ulster Cancer Foundation
40–42 Eglantine Avenue
Belfast BT9 6DX
Tel: 0232 663281

Provides information over the phone about all aspects of cancer.

Westminster Pastoral Foundation
23 Kensington Square
London W8 5HN
Tel: 01-937 6956

Offers counselling for a wide variety of personal or family problems. Has affiliated centres in other parts of the country.

WACC! (Women Against Cervical Cancer)
4 Grosvenor Cottages
Eaton Terrace
London SW1 8NA

Women's Health Concern
Ground Floor
17 Earls Terrace
London W8 6LP
Tel: 01-602 6669

Leaflets and information.

Women's Health and Reproductive Rights Information Centre
52 Featherstone Street
London EC1Y 8RT

Tel: 01-251 6580 (Mon, Tues, Thurs, Fri 12.00–4.00
Wed 2.00–6.00)

Women & Medical Practice
666 High Road
Tottenham
London N17
Tel: 01-885 2277

Health information and counselling for women.

Women's National Cancer Control Campaign (WNCCC)
1 South Audley Street
London W1Y 5DQ
Tel: 01-499 7532/3/4
    01-495 4995 (Helpline)

Provides information and advice on breast self-examination, screening and early detection of cancer of the breast and cervix. Provides help and advice for women going through the process of diagnosis and treatment.

Yorkshire Regional Cancer Organisation (YRCO)
Cookridge Hospital
Leeds LS16 6QB
Tel: 0532 673411 Ext. 406

Further reading

Cancer: A Family Doctor Booklet, Chris Williams. Family Doctor Publications, 1988.

Cancer: A Guide for Patients and Their Families, Chris and Sue Williams. Wiley, 1986.

Cancer: What It Is and How It Is Treated, H. Smedley, K. Sikora and R. Stepney. Basil Blackwell, 1986.

Coping with Cancer: Making Sense of it All, Rachael Clyne. Thorsons, 1986.

Living with Cancer, Jenny Bryan and Joanne Lyall. Penguin, 1987.

Understanding Cancer, Which Guide. Consumers Association, 1986.

Cancer and Emotion: Psychological Preludes and Reactions to Cancer, Jennifer Hughes. Wiley, 1987.

A Short History of Breast Cancer, Daniel de Moulin. Martinus Nijhoff, 1983.

Breast Cancer: The Facts, Michael Baum (new edn). Oxford University Press, 1988.

A Woman's Guide to Breast Health, Cath Cirket. Grapevine, 1989.

Your Smear Test, Graham H. Barker, FRCS, MRCOG. Adamson Books, 1987.

Prevention of Cervical Cancer: The Patient's View, Tina Posner and Martin Vessey. King Edward's Hospital Fund for London, 1988.

Cervical Cancer and How to Stop Worrying About it, Judith Harvey, Sue Mack and Julian Woolfson. Faber & Faber, 1988.

Cervical Smear Test: What Every Woman Should Know, Albert Singer, FRCOG and Dr Anne Szarewski. Positive Health Guides, 1988.

Positive Smear, Susan Quilliam. Penguin, 1989.

Women on Hysterectomy, Anne Dickson and Nikki Henriques. Thorsons, 1986.

Beating the Ladykillers: Women and Smoking, Bobbie Jacobson. Pluto, 1986.

Evening Star, Dea Trier Morch. Serpent's Tail, 1988.

Anatomy of an Illness: As Perceived by the Patient, Norman Cousins. Bantam, 1981.

In The Company of Others, Jory Graham. Victor Gollancz, 1983.

Love, Medicine and Miracles, Bernie S. Siegel. Rider, 1988.

Getting Well Again, O. Carl Simonton, MD, Stephanie Matthews-Simonton, James L. Creighton. Bantam.

The Handbook of Complementary Medicine, Stephen Fulder. Coronet, 1984.

The Bristol Programme, Penny Brohn. Century, 1987.

A Gentle Way With Cancer: What Every Patient Should Know about the Therapies which can Influence the Fight for Recovery, Brenda Kidman. Century Arrow, 1986.

New Approaches to Cancer: What Everyone Needs to Know about Orthodox and Complementary Methods for Prevention, Treatment and Cure. Shirley Harrison, Century Paperbacks, 1987.

A Time to Heal, Beata Bishop. Severn House, 1985.

The Bitter Pill, Dr Ellen Grant. Corgi, 1986.

Whose Body Is It? The Troubling Issue of Informed Consent, Carolyn Faulder. Virago, 1985.

I Don't Know What to Say: How to Help and Support Someone Who is Dying, Robert Buckman. Papermac, 1988.

To Do No Harm: DES and the Dilemmas of Modern Medicine, Roberta J. Apfel and Susan M. Fisher. Yale University Press, 1984.

Thorsons Guide to Medical Tests, Joanna Trevelyan and Dr David Dowson with Ruth West. Thorsons, 1989.

The Wound and the Doctor, Glin Bennett. Secker & Warburg, 1987.

More Difficult Exercises, Diana Moran. Bloomsbury, 1989.

Index